Pocket Guide
for
Healthcare

Tools for the Elimination of Waste in Hospitals, Clinics, and Physician Group Practices

Todd Sperl
Rob Ptacek
Jayant Trewn, PhD

ISBN 978-0-9898030-0-7

MCS Media, Inc. (The Lean Store)
888 Ridge Road
Chelsea, MI 48118
United States of America
Telephone 734-475-4301

Cover concept and art direction: Erika Humke
Page design: Janice McKinley

Library of Congress Cataloging-in-Publication Data

This publication is designed to provide the most up-to-date, accurate and authoritative information for the improvement of business processes and practices. It is sold with the understanding that neither the authors, editors, nor the publisher are engaged in providing legal, accounting, or other professional service. If legal advice or other expert assistance is required, the services of a competent professional consultant should be sought.

All MCS Media, Inc. books are available at special quantity discounts to use as sales promotions, corporate training programs, and/or any other avenue conveying information on continuous improvement.

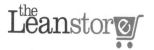

Message to Lean Senseis, Six Sigma Belts, Continuous Improvement Specialists, and Change Agents

This book bridges the gap between a highly quantitative analysis of a process that requires extensive training (i.e., Six Sigma certification) and a more simplified approach that can be used and understood by the masses (i.e., Lean thinking). The goal of this book is to make the methods and tools of Lean and Six Sigma accessible to more people and provide a common sense or "practical" approach to problem solving and continuous improvement. This book is intended to be used by Sigma Belt Levels, Lean Senseis (i.e., teachers), Continuous Improvement Specialists, front-line managers, and supervisors of departments and work groups, and improvement team members in their efforts to improve the patient care experience while reducing waste and variation in all types of healthcare processes. The Lean Six Sigma tools and concepts are presented relative to the A3 Report to provide a definitive how-to guide to problem solving and continuous improvement (Kaizen) initiatives.

The examples contained in this book are from a wide range of hospitals, clinics, and physician group practices, and will assist team members to fully understand the tool's usage and purpose. The following are the healthcare organizations we wish to recognize for their contributions:

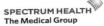

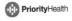

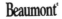

Throughout this book, the different improvement methodologies that organizations may already be using to meet the Joint Commission requirements are recognized and mentioned. We acknowledge that all have their benefits. It is important to select the one that fits the organization and will be widely used. The methodology should be easy to understand and follow, therefore better engaging the employees, as well as providing a visual management structure for reporting and sustaining continuous improvement initiatives. We will be referring to the familiar Six Sigma methodology of Define-Measure-Analyze-Improve-Control (or D-M-A-I-C) throughout this publication.

The examples provided throughout this publication demonstrate how a Lean or Six Sigma tool was used in a particular setting. We have presented them in this manner to provide a general understanding on how the tools can be applied in everyday (i.e., practical) healthcare services. This includes supporting key parts of the Affordable Care Act (such as EMR deployment and meaningful use) and the IHI Triple Aim initiative.

Moving forward, we will be referring to the patient as the customer in many situations. It is acknowledged that situations will vary greatly in healthcare. In some projects the customer may be the physician, lab tech, dietician, insurance or drug rep, etc., but ultimately, in the end, the customer will be the patient. We expect with the knowledge conveyed in this book, as well as the experiences from your improvement projects, that one day you will become a Lean "Sensei."

Our sincere thanks go to Debra Williams, Chief Nursing Officer, for her input and review of this publication.

The sister publication Practical Lean Six Sigma for Healthcare organizes the tools and examples in the healthcare familiar Assess, Diagnosis, Treat, and Prevent model of patient care. For this smaller, pocket guide version we have chosen the Six Sigma D-M-A-I-C methodology for organizing the same tools and examples.

The Practical Lean Six Sigma for Healthcare Series of apps is now available on various emerging technology platforms such as the iPad, Android, and Windows tablets. The Practical Lean Six Sigma for Healthcare Series presents the full spectrum of Lean thinking and its applications to healthcare with assessments, tools, case study examples, Sensei tips, and practical forms and worksheets to support your continuous improvement initiatives. Visit the iTunes App Store as well as other social media outlets.

Table of Contents

Publisher's Message

Looking for the latest and greatest methods or ideas in continuous improvement in healthcare? Google "Lean healthcare," "Lean production," "continuous improvement in healthcare," "Six Sigma healthcare," or "Lean Sigma healthcare" etc. and you will have pages and pages of links to solutions and promises to improve patient care and safety while reducing costs from a wide variety of educational institutions, non-profit and healthcare services organizations, and consultants. Or, maybe you just want to find resources available that will enhance your current program. In either situation, this can be overwhelming. "Continuous improvement methodologies," "Lean healthcare," or "Lean Sigma healthcare" etc. boils down to a simple process of identifying and eliminating waste and variation through Total Employee Involvement (TEI) while improving the patient care experience.

Authors and practitioners have contributed their successes of Lean and Six Sigma in nearly every industry segment via books, conferences, blogs, tweets, and other social media outlets. We would like to thank them for their contributions. Even though the Lean Six Sigma tools and the structured methodology discussed in this book may be similar, we believe the practical approach using examples from a wide range healthcare facility types and functions within, definitive how-to steps, Sensei Tips (from the authors with over 25 years of Lean Sigma experience in healthcare), and Lean Thinking Statements will enlighten managers, team leaders, supervisors, and front-line employees to an integrated and standard problem solving and continuous improvement approach. This will assist in reducing costs and all forms of wastes in hospitals, clinics, and physician group practices by providing guidance with the proper selection (and use) of Lean and Six Sigma tools, all within a standard improvement protocol and A3 reporting format.

Lean and Six Sigma, referenced as Lean Sigma for brevity throughout this publication, is no longer a tool to gain a competitive advantage rather a key success factor. That is, Lean (and Six Sigma) is one of those factors that you better have in your business or you will not be in business.

Don Tapping

> *Perfection is not obtainable. But if we chase perfection, we can catch excellence.*
> Vince Lombardi

Sensei Thoughts Before Beginning Your Journey

These past few years have brought EMRs, Meaningful Use, Accountable Care Organizations, Value Based Purchasing (Patient Satisfaction Surveys, Patient Centered Medical Home, etc.), and Performance Based Financial Penalties (Hospital Readmission, infection rates, etc.). These all come with challenges that require a new way of doing business. Therefore, as you read this book, keep in mind that each project (i.e., challenge) uses a variety of Lean Sigma tools. No project will require every tool listed in this book or that the same tools be applied in exactly the same order. However, if you follow a structured methodology and use the A3 Project Report format, you will find projects become easier - especially as employees understand, learn, and experience success. *The A3 Project Report is designed to help you "tell the story" in a logical and visual way and act as a road map for continuous improvement and problem solving initiatives.* As your familiarity and experience increases, so will your ability to effectively select the appropriate tools.

A skill requirement that crosses all environments and situations is the ability to effectively manage and lead change. Technology, governmental regulations, patient's demand for quality and efficient services, constrained resources etc. will constantly require that organizations improve their processes and with that comes change. The first chapter, Managing Change, is well-positioned for being a key success factor to understand while moving forward with any type of a Lean Six Sigma approach and improvement methodology.

Improvement projects are comprised of many mini-solutions that will require people to adapt to change. For employees to be part of the change process, effective communication and Total Employee Involvement (TEI) must be present, as well as employees must be treated with dignity and respect. By using the knowledge, tools, and concepts conveyed in this book, as well as ensuring that the "people-side" is addressed by applying the principles contained in *Today's Lean Leader* book, will a continuous improvement or problem solving project be successful. *Project success does not just happen!*

Note: All the forms, worksheets, charts, graphs, etc. described in this book can be easily created in Microsoft Office (Word, Excel, etc.) or as active pdfs. Your Electronic Medical Records system may also contain similar forms that can be customized. They can also be obtained at www.TheLeanStore.com under the Healthcare section of eTools.

Author's Bios

Todd Sperl

Todd Sperl is an enthusiastic, creative speaker and process improvement expert who looks beyond today's problems to find tomorrow's solutions. As Owner and Managing Partner of Lean Fox Solutions, Todd's vision is to improve the patient care experience from one healthcare touch point to the next. As a Master Black Belt and Lean Sensei, Todd's exceptional track record of process improvement has been based on his philosophy of total enterprise engagement in change. Todd received his BS in Psychology from the University of Wisconsin-River Falls and an MS in Industrial-Organizational Psychology from St. Mary's University in San Antonio, Texas. Todd can be contacted at tsperl@leanfoxsolutions.com or visit www.leanfoxsolutions.com.

Rob Ptacek

Rob Ptacek is a Partner in the Global Lean Institute and President and CEO of Competitive Edge Training and Consulting, a firm specializing in leader and organizational development, and Lean Enterprise transformations. Rob holds a BS in Metallurgical Engineering from Michigan Technological University and a Masters of Management from Aquinas College. Rob has held leadership positions in Quality, Sales, and Operations Management, and has over 25 years of practical experience implementing continuous improvements in a variety of industries. Rob can be contacted at ptacek@i2k.com.

Jayant Trewn, PhD

Jayant Trewn is an Industrial Engineer specializing in Quality Systems design, development, implementation, and management. Jayant has accumulated over a decade of experience working in healthcare organizations such as Spectrum Health Medical Group, Beaumont Hospitals, and Lason Systems where he built healthcare delivery process improvement programs based on Lean, Six Sigma, and PDCA concepts. Jayant has authored the book *Multivariate Statistical Methods in Quality Engineering* and he has been published in international journals. He holds a Doctorate degree in Industrial Engineering from the College of Engineering, Wayne State University, Detroit, MI, USA. He earned his MBA in Information Systems at Wayne State University and his Bachelor of Engineering degree from Madras University, India. Jayant can be contacted at jtrewn@leanfoxsolutions.com.

How to Use *The Practical Lean Six Sigma Pocket Guide for Healthcare*

The Practical Lean Six Sigma Pocket Guide for Healthcare is designed as a convenient, quick reference, and, most importantly, a step-by-step implementation guide. You can put your finger on any tool within a matter of seconds! Use the book as follows:

- ❖ Navigate the Prepare - Define - Measure - Analyze - Improve - Control right side book tabs.
- ❖ Complete the A3 Project Report as you learn and apply the various tools on the project by:
  1. Go to the tab in the book that corresponds to the D-M-A-I-C Phase you are working on.
  2. Read about the tools for that phase of your project.
  3. Apply the appropriate tools.
  4. Complete the relevant section of the A3 Project Report.
  5. Repeat 1 - 4 as you navigate through the phases and complete your project.
- ❖ Use the Case Study Example Look-Ahead and Tool Grid Matrix to direct you to specific pages with examples or case studies for hospitals, clinics, and/or physician group practices.
- ❖ Use the Index for quick access to a specific topic or tool.

The tools are presented in the logical order relative to the D - M - A - I - C Phases and A3 (Project) Report format; keep in mind that many tools can be used repeatedly across the phases. For example, the value stream map introduced in the Define Phase and A3 Report - 2. Current State will most likely be used in the Improve Phase and A3 Report - 5. Future State; the Run Chart introduced in the Analyze Phase will most likely be used (or updated) in the Control Phase, and so forth.

The Lean Sigma journey is similar to the treatment of a patient. It requires people (healthcare providers and staff) and support from various departments and ancillary staff to effectively apply the concepts and tools. Just as patient treatment is individually tailored, so must improvement tools be tailored to the facility, department, and/or process in which they will be used.

The following icons of Assess, Diagnosis, Treat, and Prevent, the common patient treatment protocol, will be your navigator throughout this book to assist with you with learning a particular topic. Also, each phase will reference the appropriate section of the A3 Project Report.

 Assess - This is the most critical step in Lean Sigma for healthcare. In medicine, professional skills are used to assess and evaluate a patient. Assessment involves teamwork represented by the icon of team members reviewing a productivity measurement. Each member of the team plays a vital role, bringing to the table different knowledge and skills. *In reference to a section in this book,* expect a brief description of the tool.

 Diagnosis - A stethoscope, EKG, lab results, etc. are used to diagnosis a patient. Using a multi-disciplinary (i.e., cross-functional team) approach allows a statement or conclusion to be drawn concerning the nature or cause requiring attention. *In reference to a section in this book,* expect information on what this tool will do as well as a thorough explanation of the tool's purpose.

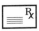 **Treat** - The prescription pad represents treatment after the Assess and Diagnosis have been completed. In medicine, the ultimate goal is to achieve wellness for a patient. *In reference to a section in this book,* you will find detailed steps or guidelines and the benefits of the tool. Treatment involves the application of a Lean Sigma tool to a process or area to attain a standardized process used as a base for continuous improvement, free of waste, error, and variation (i.e., a state of process wellness).

 Prevent - "An apple a day keeps the doctor away." This implies preventing illness and sustaining health. In healthcare, prevention is the key to the ultimate goal of wellness. *In reference to a section in this book,* you will find Sensei Tips, which include case studies, example worksheets, and actual photos conveying successful applications of that particular tool or concept from a Lean Sensei's experience. These examples are from hospitals, clinics, and physician group practices in North America (U.S. and Canada).

Note: We have kept this book relatively statistics-free. There are times when more statistical analyses are required in your project. If so, please consult additional materials or resources (e.g., Six Sigma Black Belt, Lean Sensei, or your quality department).

What is Lean?

Lean is a never-ending, systematic approach for identifying and eliminating waste and improving flow of a process while engaging employees. Lean is a way of thinking that can easily be applied to every type of organization. The entire focus of Lean is customer-driven; it is the customer who determines the value and the amount they are willing to pay for the product or service.

There are three reasons why Lean can be used with confidence.

1. **The training requirements and implementation time for Lean are minimal.** Basic concepts of Lean can be taught very quickly and improvements can be implemented the same day. For example, when an individual understands that some of their daily activities are non value-added or waste (activities such as excess time spent walking, waiting, and moving), immediate changes can be made to improve the process. Waste reduction becomes automatic for people as they become aware of waste. Improvements are continuously made at all stages of work. Often, the completion of one improvement stimulates the participants to think of other areas for improvement.

2. **The application of Lean improvement in an organization is broad.** In Lean, tools such as 5S can get everyone engaged fairly quickly and easily with no additional resources required. 5S stands for Sort, Set-In-Order, Shine, Standardize, and Sustain. It is a program that improves the efficiencies of having resources (supplies, equipment, information, etc.) in the right place at the right time and ready to use.

3. **Improvements made using Lean concepts, commonly referred to as Kaizen, positively impact other areas of the organization as well as the bottom-line.** Customers are more satisfied with decreased wait times, reduction of duplicate documentation, and fewer errors or mix-ups. In Lean, employees are encouraged and empowered to improve their work processes.

Lean, the Toyota Production System, waste elimination, and continuous improvement are used synonymously, all with the similar objective of improving the patient care experience. A phrase from Toyota that summarizes Lean is *"At Toyota we get brilliant results from average people managing a brilliant process. Others get average results from brilliant people managing broken processes."*

What is Six Sigma?

Six Sigma is a statistical term. Six Sigma measures how much of the normal process variation (operational width) falls within the process requirements (specification width). Sigma (σ) measures the variation or "spread" of a process. *Six Sigma, as a business tool or project methodology, is a structured, quantitative, five phase approach to continuous improvement and problem solving.* The five phases are: Define - Measure - Analyze - Improve - Control and are commonly referred to as the D-M-A-I-C process (or phases).

The term Six is the number of sigmas (standard deviations) as a measure from the mean in a bell-shaped normal distribution curve, as shown below:

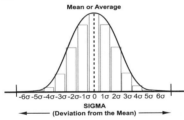

Mean or Average

-6σ -5σ -4σ -3σ -2σ -1σ 0 1σ 2σ 3σ 4σ 5σ 6σ

SIGMA
← (Deviation from the Mean) →

The goal of Six Sigma is to eliminate defects and minimize variability. In statistical terms, if an organization, department, or process achieves a Six Sigma level of performance, 99.99966% of its process outputs are defect-free and meet expectations. In other words, that organization, department, or process will have no more than 3.4 defects per million opportunities (of errors). The table below summarizes the sigma or variation level and error (or defect) rate per million opportunities (DPMO):

Process Capability or Sigma Level	Defects (or Errors) Per Million Opportunities (DPMO)	Percent Acceptable (or Error Free)
6 σ	3.4	99.99966%
5 σ	233	99.9767%
4 σ	6,210	99.379%
3 σ	66,807	93.32%
2 σ	308,538	69.15%
1 σ	691,462	30.9%

Six Sigma forces organizations to pursue perfection by asking if 99% acceptability is good enough. If 99% acceptable is good enough, consider the following:

Sigma	Patient Personal Items	Coding Processing	Scheduling Time	DPMO	% Yield
3σ	3,660 Patients With Misplaced Personal Items **Every Day**	770 Coding Errors **Every Day** Require Correction	257 Calls **Each Day** Exceed The Two Minute On-Hold Time	66,800	93.32000%
4σ	340 Patients With Misplaced Personal Items **Every Day**	72 Coding Errors **Every Day** Require Correction	24 Calls **Each Day** Exceed The Two Minute On-Hold Time	6,210	99.3790%
5σ	12 Patients With Misplaced Personal Items **Every Day**	13 Coding Errors **Every Day** Require Correction	5 Calls **Each Week** Exceed The Two Minute On-Hold Time	230	99.97700%
6σ	6 Patients With Misplaced Personal Items **Every Month**	**During The Year**, Only 10 Coding Errors Require Correction	**During The Year**, 3 Calls Exceed The Two Minute On-Hold Time	3.4	99.99966%

The following Sigma Level Versus Defects chart highlights the sigma levels for three broad categories of organizations as well as common healthcare processes:

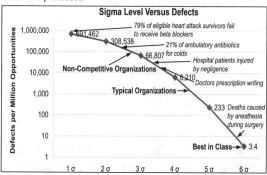

Note: Aim for standard, waste-free processes (i.e., low hanging fruit removed) before introducing Six Sigma initiatives. We have seen successes when healthcare process improvement initiatives begin with a Lean approach to remove waste and introduce standardization. Subsequently, followed by the introduction of Six Sigma to improve reliability, reduce variability, and eliminate defects/errors.

What is Lean Six Sigma for Healthcare?

Lean Six Sigma (or *Lean Sigma*) is the combination of customer-focused and waste elimination efforts of Lean with the quantitative analysis and structured D-M-A-I-C methodology of Six Sigma. Lean Sigma can be, and is for many organizations, a very powerful business improvement tool. It systematically blends the best of the two approaches to eliminate all waste (i.e., non value-added activities) and variation from a process which subsequently lowers the cost and improves the quality of the process. In the healthcare industry, Lean Sigma allows organizations that aggressively adopt these practices to remain competitive, develop a cross-trained workforce, establish a safe workplace free of errors and process variation, and heal patients in a cost-effective manner.

Lean Sigma tools are used to:

❖ Improve physician, staff, and patient satisfaction
❖ Identify and eliminate waste quickly and efficiently
❖ Increase communication and speed of services and information at all levels of the organization
❖ Reduce costs, improve quality, and meet obligations of a product or service in a safe environment
❖ Initiate improvement activities and empower employees to make improvements themselves
❖ Track and monitor to control improvements to ensure sustainability
❖ Implement and manage change with a systematic mind set

Lean Sigma is truly a compilation of world-class practices. What you will begin to see when you understand and work with these tools is a renewed management philosophy that continues to embrace those values of improved patient safety, quality of care, patient and staff satisfaction, and patient access to care.

Lean Six Sigma Philosophies and Principles

A solid foundation stems from understanding and practicing Lean Sigma Philosophies. The philosophies of a continuous (relentless) elimination of waste and non value-added activities in everything we do and the conservation of all resources at every level of operation are key to a successful Lean Sigma transformation. Additionally, Lean Sigma philosophy calls for the simplification of all tasks and efforts to eliminate process variation and improve flow. Absolute perfection is the goal. Very few organizations embrace Lean Sigma at this level. Lean management principles have been used effectively in manufacturing companies for decades, particularly in Japan.

Creating this foundation of Philosophies and Principles will ensure the required support is available as additional efforts in Lean and Six Sigma Concepts are applied through the use of Lean Sigma Tools.

Over the past decade, Lean Sigma Philosophies and Principles have been adopted by healthcare. Although healthcare differs in many ways from manufacturing, there are surprising similarities whether building a car or providing healthcare for a patient. Healthcare workers at all levels must rely on multiple, complex processes to accomplish their tasks and provide value to the customer (i.e., patient). By working to eliminate waste (Lean) and reduce variability (Six Sigma) healthcare systems have reduced costs and improved patient satisfaction scores.

These building blocks are illustrated in the diagram below. Starting with a strong foundation of Lean Sigma Philosophies and Lean Sigma Principles, these building blocks are used to support the Lean and Six Sigma Concept pillars providing patients with Access to Care with Improved Patient Safety, Enhanced Quality, Efficient Operations, and Cost Effective Services.

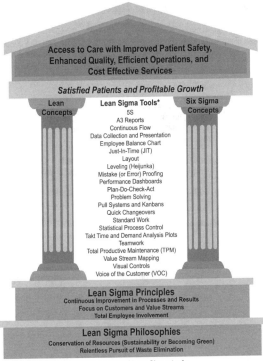

Access to Care with Improved Patient Safety, Enhanced Quality, Efficient Operations, and Cost Effective Services

Satisfied Patients and Profitable Growth

Lean Concepts

Six Sigma Concepts

Lean Sigma Tools*

5S
A3 Reports
Continuous Flow
Data Collection and Presentation
Employee Balance Chart
Just-In-Time (JIT)
Layout
Leveling (Heijunka)
Mistake (or Error) Proofing
Performance Dashboards
Plan-Do-Check-Act
Problem Solving
Pull Systems and Kanbans
Quick Changeovers
Standard Work
Statistical Process Control
Takt Time and Demand Analysis Plots
Teamwork
Total Productive Maintenance (TPM)
Value Stream Mapping
Visual Controls
Voice of the Customer (VOC)

Lean Sigma Principles
Continuous Improvement in Processes and Results
Focus on Customers and Value Streams
Total Employee Involvement

Lean Sigma Philosophies
Conservation of Resources (Sustainability or Becoming Green)
Relentless Pursuit of Waste Elimination

* Not all inclusive of Lean Sigma tools

Lean Sigma Philosophies

The Lean Sigma Philosophies must exist as the solid foundation for a Lean Sigma transformation. The two main Lean Sigma Philosophies are:

1. Conservation of Resources (Sustainability or Becoming Green)
2. Relentless Pursuit of Waste Elimination

Understanding these Lean Sigma Philosophies and applying the Lean Sigma Principles (next section) will help drive a Lean Sigma transformation. It is essential that employees at all levels of the organization be made aware of these Lean Sigma Philosophies.

Lean Sigma Principles

Lean Sigma Principles must also be present for transformations. They provide the unchanging, solid foundation to build and improve upon. The three key Lean Sigma Principles, supported by Lean Sigma Philosophies, are:

1. Continuous Improvement in Processes and Results – Do not focus *only* on the results or bottom-line. Instead, focus on processes that deliver consistent, waste-free results.
2. Focus on Customers and Value Streams – Focus on the entire process, from the customer pull or demand to demand fulfillment and customer satisfaction. Focus on how materials, information, or service requests flow through a process.
3. Total Employee Involvement – Organization leaders must make it safe and as easy as possible for people to engage in improvement activities.

Creating this foundation of Philosophies and Principles will require that management support this endeavor by making employee training robust, being sincerely involved when and where practical, and letting those closest to the process be involved in any change.

Six Sigma Concepts and Lean Concepts

The Six Sigma Concepts are:

- ❖ Scientific Method
- ❖ Statistical Methods
- ❖ Focus on Variation
- ❖ Proven Methodology
- ❖ Look for Hidden Wastes
- ❖ D-M-A-I-C
- ❖ Quantitative Analysis
- ❖ Voice of the Customer
- ❖ Zero Defects
- ❖ Common Goal of Six Sigma

The Lean Concepts are:

- ❖ Value and Waste
- ❖ Quality First
- ❖ Speak with Data and Facts
- ❖ Customer Focus
- ❖ Total Employee Involvement
- ❖ Plan-Do-Check-Act
- ❖ Flow
- ❖ Waste Elimination
- ❖ Performance Measures

The overall goal of a Lean Sigma transformation is to understand, identify, and then eliminate (or reduce) waste. The following are the twelve wastes and are also referred to as The Dirty Dozen:

1. Overproduction
2. Inventory or Work In Process (WIP)
3. Waiting or Delays
4. Motion
5. Transport
6. Defects or Errors
7. Overprocessing
8. Skills and Knowledge
9. Unevenness
10. Overburden
11. Environmental Resources
12. Social Responsibility

For a detailed explanation of wastes, consider purchasing the book, *Today's Lean! Learning About and Identifying Waste* available at www. TheLeanStore.com or review the *Waste Walk* section in the *Measure Phase* of this book.

Note: Healthcare is data rich but information poor. For example, communication is still a challenge among hospitals, physician group practices, specialists, and patients. There is a lack of standards in collecting data, which leads to poor or misused information. A Lean Six Sigma approach using the A3 Project Report format with the D-M-A-I-C (or similar methodology) will allow the data collection (and processes) to be standardized across platforms, thereby allowing "useful" information to be obtained and used that will have a notable impact on the patient care experience.

Engaging Today's Workforce

Improving patient access to care and improving patient and staff satisfaction will lead to overall organizational growth and profitability. Growth and profitability are essential for any organization to survive. Through implementing a Lean Sigma transformation, a business is more likely to survive, become stronger, and will be able to provide wage and earnings growth, and advancement in a safer, more stable work environment. But at the heart of any Lean Sigma transformation is understanding your people (i.e., specifically the generations in today's workforce) and engaging them to take a more pro-active role in all problem solving and continuous improvement efforts.

There are four generations in the workforce today interacting on a day-to-day basis, each with different computer skills and work experiences. These differences, if not acknowledged and leveraged appropriately, can give rise to frustration, conflict, and misinterpretation – all of which can contribute to a non-Lean Sigma work environment. However, use each generation's positive work styles (i.e., technical and work experience skills) to foster a more creative and diverse atmosphere. It is imperative for managers and front-line workers to understand generational and skill-set differences. Work to improve communications between these generations ultimately improves the quality of decision-making as well as improves the flow of information, products, services, etc. throughout the organization. It is imperative not to underestimate the importance of people's attitudes and how they can impact work processes within an organization.

The years that differentiate the generations in today's workforce, as outlined in this section, may be defined a bit differently due to a certain set of criteria used by various organizations. Keep in mind the bigger picture of the "groups" of people as a generation; these are generalizations. We do not mean to "categorize" a certain age group in any negative way. The intent is to recognize the differences that do exist and use those differences, along with the right balance of technology, to improve an organization's communication.

The following are the four working generations and some general attributes of each that exist in today's workforce (years and numbers referenced are for the United States):

The **Matures (Traditionalist, Veterans, and Silent) Generation** is the oldest generation in the workforce and these people were born between 1925 and 1945. There are approximately 63.2 million Matures in the workforce. The Matures are currently retiring or facing retirement in the next few years. This group was largely defined by their experiences in the Great Depression (1929) and in World War II (1941 – 1945).

- ❖ Value: respect for authorities, conformity, and discipline
- ❖ Key Word: loyal
- ❖ Their families are very traditional (nuclear)
- ❖ Education is typically seen as a dream
- ❖ Communicate in person (i.e., face-to-face)
- ❖ Deal with money by saving it, and when spent, paying with cash

The **Baby Boomer Generation** is the second oldest generation in the workforce, and these people were born between 1946 and 1964. There are roughly 76.8 million Baby Boomers in the workforce. The Baby Boomers are currently becoming empty nesters (i.e., having no children at home) and make up the largest segment in the workforce. These people grew up post World War II and have experienced Kennedy's Camelot years at the White House, Woodstock, and the Vietnam War.

- ❖ Value: being involved
- ❖ Key Word: optimistic
- ❖ Their family is disintegrating (divorce rates beginning to increase dramatically)
- ❖ Education is a birthright
- ❖ Communicate by phone and liked to be called at anytime
- ❖ Deal with money by buying something now and paying for it later

The **Generation Xers** are the people born between 1965 and 1980. There are roughly 52.4 million Gen Xers in the workforce. These people are buying, if they can afford it, their first homes, waiting longer to start families, and beginning to move to higher-level management positions being vacated by the Matures and Baby Boomers. These people grew up in the decade after the Cold War and during the fall of the Berlin Wall.

- ❖ Value: fun and informality
- ❖ Key Word: skepticism
- ❖ Family is noticing latchkey kids (children being left alone at home while parents are at work)
- ❖ See education as a way to get some place in life
- ❖ Communicate with cell phones and like to be called only when at work
- ❖ Deal with money by saving, conserving, and being cautious

The **Generation Y (Millenials)** are the youngest working generation in the workforce and these people are born between 1981 and 1999. There are roughly 7.6 million Millenials in the workforce now, with many more on the way. These people are facing independence and moving out of their parent's homes after completing college and entering the workforce while seeking further academic degrees.

- ❖ Value: confidence, extreme fun, and being social
- ❖ Key Word: realistic
- ❖ Families are typically merged
- ❖ Education is seen as an incredible expense
- ❖ Communicate using text messaging and smart devices
- ❖ Deal with money by earning it and then spending it

The following Pie Chart summarizes the current breakdown of workers in the U.S. workforce as of 2010:

U.S. Population of Generations in the Workforce (2010)

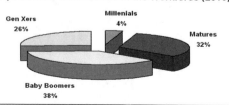

Gen Xers 26%

Millenials 4%

Matures 32%

Baby Boomers 38%

The emerging workforce born after 1999 is referred to as the **"Cyber Generation."** This group of young people is still in elementary and high schools and soon will have a profound effect on work environments and customer expectations. The potential number of workers in the Cyber Generation rival that of the Baby Boomer generation, yet their childhood influences will be quite different. The Cyber Generation will have spent their entire lives with the constant availability and bombardment of real-time news, videos, communication, social-cyber interaction, and instant information and gratification. This group has watched military conflicts and world crisis unfold in near real-time and will expect the same of their business interactions and buying habits. As workers and consumers, their demands will far exceed those of any previous generation and their respect for conformance and red tape will be intolerable. Some qualities of this generation are:

- ❖ Never lived without an internet connection
- ❖ Never lived without a cell phone with instant text or messaging
- ❖ Never lived without laptops and tablets
- ❖ Angry and or feel helpless when out of communications
- ❖ YouTube and Wikipedia providing instant learning opportunities at their finger tips
- ❖ Socially connected instantly
- ❖ Constant detailed world event news available
- ❖ Use of Facebook, FaceTime, Skype, Twitter, LinkedIn, tablets, email, etc.
- ❖ Fear of loss of social contact
- ❖ Reality and social television on demand

The mix of workers in the workforce will be a changing dynamic, and leaders must continually adapt their strategy to achieve success.

Understanding workplace communication, generational similarities and differences, and employee motivation will help foster an environment necessary to identify and eliminate waste. The 10 Tips to Help Bridge the Socio – Techno Gap are:

1. *Communicate early and often.* All generations have a need to be included in any change; however, it is acknowledged that there are times when everyone cannot be part of the team that is initiating or designing the change. If that is the case, ensure communication from the manager is done early in the process as well as provide regular updates. It is suggested that updates be provided online. Mistakes or reasons why things do not get completed on time may be due to miscommunication in the workplace.

2. **Be enlightening.** Show how diversity can benefit a company. Be positive when it comes to generational gaps and working toward eliminating the gaps. Discuss openly what could be some additional motivators for each generation. For example, the Baby Boomer employee may want additional time-off after the completion of a large project while a Generation X employee may prefer a flex-schedule to accommodate their lifestyle. Human Resources may need to be involved.

3. **Be open.** Have open conversations about the differences in generations. Share experiences and viewpoints in a safe environment. Knowing there are differences between generations is important, however, it is more important to manage these differences. When and where appropriate, have employees share work and technical experiences via the company newsletter, blog, or Intranet.

4. **Be flexible.** Create a work environment that all generations will like. If a Matures Generation employee likes title recognition then create an appropriate title. If a Baby Boomer wants a formal meeting, let that happen but limit the time to accommodate the Generation Y employees (Generation Y employees like short meetings). Utilize text messaging, smart devices, and the Internet to accommodate the younger generations communication style, but also have formal meetings to accommodate the Baby Boomers and Matures.

5. **Be creative.** Be creative in providing rewards for people. Different generational employees like different rewards, therefore, research what rewards each generation likes and accommodate accordingly. For example, the Matures and Baby Boomer Generations would most likely prefer a certificate or monogrammed company sweater than a team lunch or gift certificate.

6. **Create learning opportunities for new software applications.** Ensure there is available training for new applications. If at all possible have training made available in different platforms, such as traditional classroom, online, or self-paced. Having a learning or training opportunity on multiple platforms will not single out any particular group.

7. **Create rules and standards.** Every generation wants to know what is expected of them as well as what is acceptable and what is not acceptable in terms of communication (i.e., all emails must be returned within one business day, receiving text messages or any type messages for non-emergency reasons while at work, etc.).

8. **Create opportunities.** When at all possible, promote employee's skills within the organization as well as communicate their successes via any and all organizational bulletin boards.

9. **Understand generational differences.** Always keep in mind that the Matures and Baby Boomer Generations value active participation and want their ideas to be heard or acknowledged. However, the Gen Xers and Millenials prefer less formal meetings and do not feel the need to have everyone's ideas heard.

10. **Keep a balance.** Since these generations exist in the workforce, and as the next generation enters, try not to let one generational style dominate as that will lead to frustrated employees and managers.

Understanding the generational gaps in the workplace can be a very important ingredient when implementing any of the Lean Sigma tools. Using the previous information and adjusting communications and work assignments accordingly improves the following:

- ❖ Employee satisfaction
- ❖ Customer satisfaction
- ❖ Communication problems
- ❖ Productivity

The following are examples of waste that can be eliminated by understanding each generation. Use these as a springboard to discuss other ways your organization can reduce and eliminate similar types of wastes that exist due to not understanding generational attributes and behaviors.

Overproduction – Example: A Matures generation employee phoning a Generation X or Y associate that they just emailed them the information. The phone call is waste.

Transport – Example: Meeting with a colleague for lunch just to answer a simple question when an email or text would suffice. Walking or driving to the destination and extra time spent on this meeting is waste.

Overprocessing – Example: Having everyone attend meetings when only certain people need to be present.

People Utilization – Example: Requiring everyone to receive training on a new application or functionality, whereas, some employees may learn it on-the-job.

Not adapting and adjusting your work style to these generational issues contribute to:

❖ Lack of standardization of processes and knowledge-sharing
❖ Higher turnover among the X-Y Generation worker
❖ Lack of succession leadership

There are some overlaps with the various attributes between the generations; this is because some traits carry on for longer than one generation. For example, agreeing to hierarchy standards in companies was common in the first two generations, however, now people are becoming less interested in 'titles' and more focused on the task at hand and using people's talents given the situation, regardless of their title. Understanding these generational strengths and weaknesses in the workplace by managers and employees alike will give an organization a competitive advantage.

The following two charts summarize the generational personal and lifestyle characteristics, along with the workplace behaviors previously discussed and listed:

Workplace Behaviors				
	Matures 1925 - 1945	Baby Boomers 1946 - 1964	Gen Xers 1965 - 1980	Millenials 1981 - 1999
Work Ethic	Hard workers Dedicated to job	Workaholics Works efficiently	Eliminate the task	Whats next? Multi-taskers
Work is...	An obligation	An exciting adventure	A difficult challenge A contract	A means to an end Fulfillment
Leadership Style	Directive Command and control	Consensual Collegial	Everyone the same Challenge others Ask why	Consensual and still evolving
Interactive Style	Individual	Team player Loves meetings	Entrepreneur	Participative
Communication	Formal Memo	In person	Direct Immediate	Email, Text Messages Voicemail
Feedback and Rewards	No news is good news Satisfaction in a job well done	Does not appreciate it Money Title recognition	Sorry to interrupt but, how am I doing? Freedom	Whenever I want it, or at the push of a button Meaningful work
Messages that motivate	Your experience is respected	You are valued and needed	Do it your own way and forget the rules	Work with others who are bright and creative

Generational Personal and Lifestyle Characteristics				
	Matures 1925 - 1945	Baby Boomers 1946 - 1964	Gen Xers 1965 - 1980	Millenials 1981 - 1999
Values	Respects authority Disciplined	Optimism Involvement	Skepticism Fun times Informality	Social
Family	Traditional Nuclear	Divorce Family moving out	Latch-key kids	Merged families
Education	A dream	More plausible A right	A way to get someplace	Very expensive
Communication	One-on-one Formal memos	Touch-tone phones Call anytime	Cell phones Call at certain times	Internet iPhones, Text messages Email
Money	Save Pay cash	Buy, buy, buy and pay later	Cautious Conservative Save	Earn the money, then spend

The following chart provides guidance on how to interact with the various generations in reference to Kaizen Events:

Kaizen Event Generational Coaching Tips, Do's and Don'ts				
	Matures 1925 - 1945	Baby Boomers 1946 - 1964	Gen Xers 1965 - 1980	Millenials 1981 - 1999
Kaizen Event Coaching Tips	Encourage them to talk about their experiences	Help them feel victorious	Prove you are an authority nothing is a given	Become the provider of information
	Match your approach to a good experience	Be responsive to competition	Appear to enjoy your work	Demonstrate personal relevance, uniqueness
	Acknowledge their "rules of engagement"	Provide opportunities for more positive experiences	No hard answers	Highlight peer-to-peer examples
	Focus on quality/structure	Become a member of their team	Provide all details, options and alternatives up front	Recognize them as individuals
Do's	Allow Matures to set the "rules of engagement"	Help them use their time wisely	Put all options on the table	Offer customization - a project just for them
	Asked what has worked for them in the past - adapt	Access their comfort level with technology in advance	Be prepared to answer "why"	Offer peer level examples
	Let them define quality - fit your approach to that	Demonstrate importance of a strong team	Present yourself as an information provider	Provide information and guidance
	Use testimonials from government, business, etc.	Customize your style to their unique needs	Use their peers as testimonials	Be a coach
	Emphasize approach has worked in the past	Emphasize working w/ you will be a good experience	Appear to enjoy your work	Try to show them that work can be fun
	Respect their experience and ask about it	Communicate the long term benefits if possible	Convey this as an opportunity	Acknowledge their uniqueness
	Communicate sincerely and often	Communicate sincerely and often	Communicate sincerely and often	Communicate sincerely and often
Don'ts	Attempt to WOW them with data or newness	Assume you know or understand their needs	Try to underplay the challenge	Create a stressful environment
	Force the use technology unnecessarily	Assume technology is the solution	View questions as an implied challenge	Forget the importance of their individuality
	Ignore their experiences	Be quick to judge	Expect them to have all the answers	Tell them what to do, show or coach them
	Show indifference	Show indifference	Show indifference	Show indifference

In summary, older generations are a natural match for their younger counterparts. Older workers are rich in experience and insight, younger workers can benefit from their successes and challenges. Combining that with the younger generation's enthusiasm and technical aptitudes, organizations can immensely benefit from this interaction in any Lean Sigma transformation.

Engaging Today's Workforce

Process Improvement Models

There are several process improvement and problem solving models available. The most common are Deming's PDCA, Six Sigma's D-M-A-I-C, Lean Healthcare's Assess, Diagnosis, Treat, and Prevent, and finally Toyota's 8 Steps. All of these models are proven, successful process improvement and problem solving models. Whichever one you choose, you need to understand it, adapt it to fit organizational needs, and to stay with it. The following is a brief description.

Plan, Do, Check, Act or PDCA is one of the most well-known cycles of improvement that coordinates continuous improvement efforts. PDCA emphasizes that improvement programs must start with careful planning, result in effective action, and move again to careful planning in a continuous cycle. Dr. Deming, who is considered by many to be the father of modern quality control, popularized PDCA.

The *Six Sigma methodology of Define, Measure, Analyze, Improve, and Control or D-M-A-I-C* is a quantitative approach that emphasizes reducing the number of errors in a process by identifying variation and looking at root causes of errors. For example, what good is it to complete a process quickly if the information is entered incorrectly? Six Sigma assumes you have a data rich environment and uses that data to attain meaningful information. Successful improvement initiatives typically will begin with a Lean approach then either migrate or integrate the Six Sigma methodology to further reduce variation and improve reliability of processes.

The *Lean Healthcare cycle of Assess, Diagnosis, Treat, and Prevent or ADTP* mirrors PDCA's cycle of improvement using healthcare terminology that healthcare workers can easily relate to. This model can also be used for continuous improvement and problem solving initiatives.

Toyota's 8 Step Problem Solving Model is an evolution of PDCA because traditional PDCA was viewed as too vague for more difficult or serious business problems. The 8 steps include: 1) Clarify the Problem, 2) Breakdown the Problem, 3) Set a Target, 4) Analyze the Root Cause, 5) Develop Countermeasures, 6) See Countermeasures Through, 7) Evaluate Results and Process, and 8) Standardize and Share Success.

The following illustration provides an overview on how these various improvement and problem solving models inter-relate:

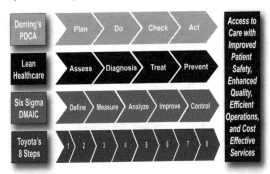

Depending on the culture and continuous improvement maturity of the organization, the availability and integrity of data, "real" involvement of top management, and available training resources will help drive which model to use. Many organizations use a hybrid model and create a blended version of their own. The important point is to choose an approach that your organization can rally around and relate to, use the A3 Project Report format (or something similar), and stick to it. In other words, standardize the continuous improvement model!

If desiring the transformation process, the organization must Prepare (next section) or "get ready" to provide the improvement team with the necessary support before applying the D-M-A-I-C Phases or any other model. The A3 Project Report along with Lean tool application within the D-M-A-I-C Phases can result in improved quality and throughput, increased customer and employee satisfaction, and be a positive impact on the bottom-line - all while leveraging *existing* resources to promote effective and efficient services.

As healthcare organizations reposition themselves to confront the daunting challenges ahead, they would be wise to remember that the major roadblocks come from people not technology - and it is a Lean philosophy of Lean thinking that helps eliminate the waste/inefficiencies to improve processes. Thus, Lean and Six Sigma are going to be an integral part of any transformation.

Case Study Example Look-Ahead and Tool Grid Matrix

The illustration on the adjacent page provides a listing of each of the topics discussed throughout this publication with reference to the type of case study or example provided. The matrix provides the following:

- ❖ An overview on the type of examples relative to a hospital, clinic, or physician group practice
- ❖ A quick reference to a specific example
- ❖ A broad perspective on how Lean can be applied in any type healthcare facility or organization

Examples are presented in the Sensei Tips at the end of each section. Some examples are specific to a hospital, clinic, or physician group practice and are noted as such. Other examples are broader in their application and relate to all three types of healthcare organizations.

All the Lean and Six Sigma tools can be applied in any of these types of organizations listed as well as long term care, rehabilitation, acute care, etc. type facilities. The practical examples provided throughout the book should assist you to apply that tool or concept in your type of facility.

Case Study Example Look-Ahead and Tool Grid Matrix

The following Tool Grid Matrix is the D-M-A-I-C model relative to the tools explained in the book. Keep in mind the overall intent of the tool and not be concerned which part of the model (or phase) it falls within. For example, Brainstorming, as it is listed in the Analyze Phase, could be used in any of the phases. This is true for many of the tools.

TOOL GRID MATRIX	PREPARE	SIX SIGMA				
Page Tool Set		DEFINE	MEASURE	ANALYZE	IMPROVE	CONTROL
2 Managing Change	•					
10 Lean Healthcare Assessment and Gap Analysis	•					
15 Stakeholder Analysis	•					
26 Project Identification	•					
31 A3 Reports	•					
36 Lean Thinking Statements for Prepare						
38 Charters		•				
42 Team Selection and Building		•				
47 Effective Meetings		•				
50 Project Management		•				
55 Value Stream and Process Maps (w/SIPOC Diagrams)		•				
70 Lean Thinking Statements for the Define Phase						
72 Waste Walk			•			
80 Value-Added versus Non Value-Added Analysis			•			
83 Constraint or Bottleneck Analysis			•			
85 Demand Analysis Plots and Takt Time			•			
90 Voice of the Customer			•			
93 Quality Function Deployment			•			
96 Measurement System Analysis (MSA)			•			
102 Process Capability			•			
106 Lean Thinking Statements for the Measure Phase						
108 Charting				•		
114 Brainstorming				•		
117 Cause and Effect (or Fishbone) Diagram				•		
119 5 Whys				•		
121 Interrelationship Diagram				•		
123 Employee Balance Chart				•		
127 Force Field Analysis				•		
129 Impact Map				•		
132 Lean Thinking Statements for the Analyze Phase						
134 Kaizen Events					•	
140 Plan-Do-Check-Act (PDCA) Process					•	
143 5S					•	
148 Visual Controls					•	
154 Mistake Proofing					•	
161 Standard Work					•	
166 Process or Work Area Layout					•	
169 Mass Customization					•	
171 Flow					•	
188 Quick Changeovers (QCO)					•	
191 Total Productive Maintenance (TPM)					•	
194 Cross-Training					•	
197 Lean Thinking Statements for the Improve Phase						
200 Statistical Process Control (SPC)						•
206 Visual Management						•
214 Standard Work for Leaders						•
221 Layered Process Audits (LPA)						•
227 Lean Thinking Statements for the Control Phase						

Prepare

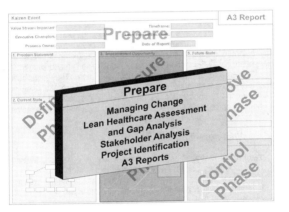

Tools listed in this section are most likely to be used at this time. All the tools can be applicable at any phase of a Kaizen Project as determined by the needs of the project team.

Managing Change

Progress is impossible without change, and those who cannot change their minds cannot change anything.
George Bernard Shaw

What is it?

Managing change is the process of how to manage the way changes in the working environment are implemented and how to lessen its effect on the workforce. It is a key topic for leaders to understand. In today's fast paced world, change and improvement are required for an organization to survive. Improper management of change and/or natural resistance to change can cripple an organization. Healthcare entities continue to face constrained resources while providing care for an aging demographic population. They have been charged with coordinating care through portals. There likely will be further efforts to consolidate, try new models of care, and leverage technology and data. As healthcare entities try to juggle all these factors at the same time, the only certainty is CHANGE.

What does it do?

Proper management of change leads to a healthy, thriving, challenging and fun work environment. Most people dread change, especially at work. At work, change means breaking with routine tasks in order to try things in a new way which forces employees out of their safety zone. This is one reason why many people are change-averse. Despite this resistance, change is necessary if a company wants to remain competitive. A good manager knows this and adapts their style of leadership and communication skills to define how the change is managed.

How do you do it?

The following steps or guidelines are used to more effectively manage change:

1. Identify the goal or what needs to be changed. Ask yourself: Is it short-term or long-term? What are the potential benefits? What are the pitfalls? Will it make the organization more competitive?

2. Help employees to understand the answers to the following three questions:

Leadership Question	Answers
Why do we need change?	Explain the business reality. Educate people as to the global marketplace, competitors, customer needs and demands, and supplier issues. Present and benchmark information and data on productivity, quality, delivery, and people measures. People can handle the truth. Define the current state.
What do we need to change?	The leaders of the organization must create a shared vision. Explain and help people understand what a productive, high quality organization looks like. Define the future state vision and what the organization is trying to become.
How do we do it together?	Leaders need a plan with regard to what methods, people, measures, and the like will be deployed to achieve the future state. Provide a systematic approach to leadership, problem solving, and improvement. Explain and educate people on the standard methods. This is what leadership is all about!

3. Identify the kind of change needed and why. Outline the specific activities that will be part of the desired change. It is best to include employees in this prior to announcing any change. Change should take place in conjunction with a plan and a schedule. It is essential for someone to be seen as the leader or advocate for change. This should be the person in charge and responsible for the change. Unplanned change can be a disaster! Anticipated and well communicated change can be stimulating.

4. Understand resistance to change. Recognize that most resistance comes from deep rooted fears of the unknown; fear of losing a job, losing pay or benefits, or status, or not being the expert, or of having to go back to school, or take a test. It is a natural human survival response. The objective is for the leader or supervisor to address peoples' fears in a positive and constructive manner. Leaders need to address people's concerns in an appropriate way. Answer questions people ask, and try to understand their concerns. In business there are no guarantees, so do not over commit. Just tell people the truth. Open and honest discussion is usually the best way to deal with resistance.

For special cases, such as an extremely vocal resistor or resistance from other leaders, leaders need to develop deliberate strategies. For vocal resistance, it may be appropriate to remove the individual(s) from the work group or team by following your organizations' performance management and disciplinary procedures.

5. Identify the specific type of change that will be required from each employee. How will their daily tasks change? Will there be additional training? How will each employee be measured in accepting the change or in their new duties?

   Change can be stressful or "painful" for organizations, but is necessary for survival.

6. Conduct a Stakeholder Analysis, if appropriate. (See *Stakeholder Analysis*)

7. Understand the managing change time line (below graph) and the following explanations for additional support and use it to identify strategies to deal with resistance.

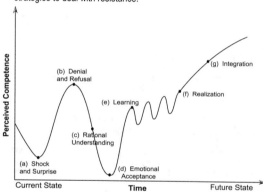

(a) Shock and Surprise - The initial knowledge of the change may be met with confrontation to unexpected situations. This can happen 'by accident' (e.g., losses in particular business units and employees must be reassigned or planned events (e.g., personal performance has been unsatisfactory and has to improve, etc.). These types of situations make people realize that their own patterns of doing things are not suitable for new conditions. Thus, their perceived own competence decreases. This stage may be met with *"I can't believe this is happening to me!"*

(b) Denial and Refusal - This would involve employees "acting out" that change is not necessary. Hence, they believe there is no need for change; their perceived competency increases again. This stage may be met with *"There is no way this change is going to happen, it's just not right!"*

(c) Rational Understanding - This is the realization that there may be a need for change; their perceived competence decreases again. Employees focus on finding short term solutions, thus they only cure symptoms. There is no willingness to change one's own patterns of behavior. This stage may be met with *"I'll go along with the change if it will get the boss off my back!"*

(d) Emotional Acceptance - This is also called the 'buy-in' phase and is the most important one. Only if management succeeds to create willingness for changing values, beliefs, and behaviors, will the organization be able to make real change happen. This stage may be met with *"It seems that it doesn't matter what I say or do!"*

(e) Learning - The new acceptance of change creates a new willingness for learning to make the best of the change. Employees start to try new behaviors and processes using the PDCA cycle. They will experience success and failure during this phase. It is the manager's task to create some early wins by starting with easier projects or providing one-on-one support with certain employees. Their perceived own competence increases. This stage may be met with *"I guess this change can't be all bad!"*

(f) Realization - Employees start to communicate in a positive way regarding the change. This communication has a feedback-effect. Employees begin to understand which behavior is effective in which situation. This, in turn, opens their minds for new experiences. Extended patterns of behavior increase organizational flexibility. Employees' perceived competency has reached a higher level than prior to change. This stage may be met with *"I can't believe I was so against this change!"*

(g) Integration - Employees totally integrate their newly acquired patterns of thinking and acting. The new behaviors become routine and the organization experiences a positive change. This stage may be met with *"I now see and understand how this change has benefited our organization and am glad to be part of it!"*

8. Assess the kind of resistance to change that may come from employees. Use the following as a guide.

- ❖ This is a hospital, not a factory!
- ❖ We already tried that.
- ❖ We walk on these floors, not eat from them.
- ❖ They (management) never tell me anything.
- ❖ They (management) don't care.
- ❖ Aren't there more 'meaty' improvements?
- ❖ Why should we spend time and money to communicate the obvious?
- ❖ We don't have time to clean up, we barely have time to get our work done!
- ❖ Our area is already spotless.
- ❖ We didn't get hired to sweep floors!
- ❖ That won't work.
- ❖ I'll wait for this to blow over.
- ❖ Silence.
- ❖ Sabotage.
- ❖ That's not my job.
- ❖ Not attending training.
- ❖ Refusing to learn something new.
- ❖ It will go away.
- ❖ We're different.
- ❖ I'm too old to change.

9. Determine a plan for each employee to accept the change in a supportive manner to help them learn and boost performance. Determine what they will need in order to accept the change. Talk to them and be yourself. Be ready to set an example by embracing and adopting the change that is also required of you.

10. Review the Managing Change Worksheet and take actions to ensure each question with a No response is addressed appropriately.

Managing Change Worksheet	
Rating System: Answer each question with a Yes or No, then focus efforts on the No responses.	**Yes or No**
1. Is there a clear and compelling reason for adopting this improvement?	
2. Is the objective data collected to convince any skeptics?	
3. Do people feel the urgency to this change?	
4. Are the motivators known for each person affected by the change?	
5. Does the senior executive team support this change?	
6. Has the proposed change been communicated with all stakeholders?	
7. Are the right people selected for the right roles?	
8. Are performance measurement and reporting systems made visible for the change?	
9. Is the training plan adequately resourced?	
10. Are project management principles and methods being used (i.e., Team Charters, Agendas, Timelines, etc.)?	
11. Is support in place ensuring transfer of training to the workplace (i.e., standards of work)?	
12. Are successes celebrated?	
13. Have we studied the changes carefully and identified if anyone is likely to lose something?	
14. Have we taken the appropriate actions to help people deal more successfully with the changes?	

The following benefits can be obtained by effectively managing change:

- ❖ Increase the likelihood for sustaining improvements
- ❖ Improve productivity
- ❖ Reduce resistance to change
- ❖ Build trust between employees and management
- ❖ Foster teamwork directly and indirectly
- ❖ Create energy
- ❖ Promote growth

Sensei Tips for Managing Change

- ❖ Recognize the cause of resistance is the fear of change.
- ❖ Answer the leading change questions; why do we need to change, what to change, what to change to, and how to do it together.
- ❖ Be honest and truthful.
- ❖ Look for subtle change resistance behaviors, and address them quickly.
- ❖ Help people understand why change is needed.
- ❖ Communicate often and early about any and all changes.
- ❖ Involve as many staff as possible in any of their processes being changed.

Case Study for Managing Change

A hospital's leadership team was concerned over recent negative trends in their emergency department, specifically, the LWOBS metric was at 2.7% and over the last three months it had been trending up, but the goal was 1.0%. Additionally, the ED's fast track and door to inpatient bed metrics were beginning to trend upward. For example, door to inpatient bed was at 4.8 hours on average, well above the goal of 3.0 hours. And treat to street (fast track) metrics were hovering at 2.4 hours on average.

The hospital's Director of Quality, Linda, suggested bringing in a Lean process improvement facilitator to further educate and teach the basic tools of Lean and Six Sigma. Most members of leadership were familiar with Lean thinking, but no one had any experience in leading a Lean project team. Linda was tasked with getting something started by the next leadership meeting; with the expectation of forming a multi-disciplinary team.

The Lean Sensei had asked Linda to invite people from various departments who coordinate care with the emergency department, including ICU/Telemetry Units, Diagnostic Imaging, Bed Control, and Respiratory Therapy to the initial session. Linda sent out the traditional email meeting notice stating that leadership required their attendance because of the LWOBS negative trend. Most of the departmental managers viewed the email as negative and accusatory.

Announcing this major and new undertaking via meeting notice and email was a mistake. The tone of the email was viewed negatively. There was initial resentment from departments to participate, which returned many defensive type questions directed to Linda. The Lean facilitator held one-on-one meetings with departmental managers to fully explain the scope and purpose of this initial meeting. Henceforth, this effective and honest communication regarding the upcoming project had the initial meeting conducted with full support of all units.

Lean Healthcare Assessment and Gap Analysis

I assess, therefore, I improve.
Don Tapping (adapted from René Decartes)

What is it?

The **Lean Healthcare Assessment and Gap Analysis** creates an understanding of what may be some potential improvement opportunities as well as provides a baseline to compare with future improvement initiatives (and subsequent assessments).

The assessment has the following five categories:

1. Leadership
2. Patient Focus
3. Process Management
4. Staff Management
5. Information and Analysis

Each section is further broken down into statements that describe qualities for each category.

What does it do?

The Lean Healthcare Assessment and Gap Analysis helps align management objectives with staff needs, desires and attitudes towards change, open communications regarding issues or problems, and provides a perspective on where the organization needs to focus resources.

Organizations use a Lean Healthcare Assessment and Gap Analysis instrument to document the current state of the entire organization, department, value stream, or key process. The assessment should be conducted at a minimum of once per year.

℞ *How do you do it?*

The following steps or guidelines are used to conduct the assessment:

1. Meet with the appropriate group that represents the process owners for each of the areas. Ensure a team-based approach is used in working through the assessment.

2. Use the following Lean Healthcare Assessment and Gap Analysis for your organization, department, value stream, or process. Each statement can be scored with the following five-level Likert item scale.

> 1 = Strongly Disagree
> 2 = Disagree
> 3 = Neither Agree nor Disagree
> 4 = Agree
> 5 = Strongly Agree

Note: The following assessment has been populated with numbers to demonstrate the charting method at the end.

Section 1 - Leadership		Score (1-5)
Vision	Leadership has defined and communicated a clear vision and is committed to process improvement.	2
Planning	Process improvement is regularly discussed at our strategic planning meetings.	1
Resources	Adequate resources are continuously assigned for achieving operational excellence (i.e., process improvements.)	2
Objectives	We have a good balance of attainable and stretch goals.	1
Accountability	We have process owners that are held accountable for performance measurements.	1
Average		**1.4**

Section 2 - Patient Focus		Score (1-5)
Listening	My organization does a good job of listening and involving its patients.	3
Measures	Patient satisfaction measurements capture actionable information needed for improvement.	3
Benchmarking	My organization obtains and uses patient information relative to competition and/or benchmarks.	2
Expectations	Patient satisfaction takes top priority at my organization.	5
Flexibility	My organization remains flexible to meet the changing expectations of the patient.	1
Equity	We practice fair and equitable business practices for our patients, providers, and clinical and operational staff.	1
Average		**2.5**

Section 3 - Process Management

		Score (1-5)
Process Focus	My organization identifies its key processes to achieve improved performance.	1
Measures	Performance measures are used for the control and improvement of key processes.	1
Efficiency	The processes that we use are smooth and work well.	1
Influence	Input from internal and external customers are incorporated into process improvement efforts.	1
Information	All necessary resources and information are available to do the work properly.	1
Variation	Process variation is understood and monitored at my organization.	1
Average		**1.0**

Section 4 - Staff Management

		Score (1-5)
Safety	Leaders demonstrate that the safety of staff is of paramount importance.	3
Training	Staff's training and development needs are openly discussed and followed through on.	2
Development	Leadership creates an encouraging and motivating environment and helps staff reach their full potential.	3
Obstacles	Staff can openly identify obstacles/problems and seek help in finding solutions.	3
Accountability	Our performance management system supports and rewards high performance.	2
Being Valued	Staff are treated as valued employees, where short and long term needs are met.	2
Average		**2.5**

Section 5 - Information and Analysis

		Score (1-5)
Information	My organization makes every effort to ensure data and information are appropriate, accurate, and reliable.	2
Monitoring	There is a system in place to monitor organizational progress against set objectives or goals.	1
Visibility	The monitoring system is clear and visible to all of the organization (e.g., scoreboards).	3
Decisions	It is clear to people how we use organizational level analysis to improve decision-making.	1
Challenge	Staff are responsible to question and/or challenge the status quo.	3
Improvement	There is an effective process to incorporate positive improvement ideas into the business plan.	2
Average		**2.0**

Note: This assessment is fairly easy to create using the Chart Wizard in Microsoft Excel. This assessment example and Radar Chart (shown in step 4) can be purchased at www.TheLeanStore.com for a nominal fee. This Assessment is also included in the Practical Lean Sigma for Healthcare Series Overview app available at the iTunes App Store and the *Practical Lean Six Sigma for Healthcare Training Set* available at TheLeanStore.com.

3. Create a Bar Chart that has the minimum value of "0" for readability. The nature of this type of assessment is that there will always be a lowest category score or individual question score.

Note: Only the Patient Focus Bar Chart is shown below:

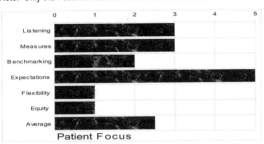

4. Create a Radar Chart to display all the results.

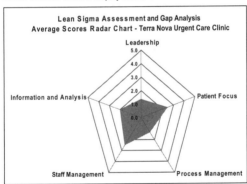

5. Use brainstorming, 5 Why Analysis, Cause and Effect Diagramming, etc. to further investigate the lower scoring areas or "gaps" in the Radar Chart. With the subsequent information from the Improvement Guide available at http://leanfoxsolutions.com/improvement-guide/ and discussion, specific improvement activities can be planned and implemented.

Sensei Tips for Lean Healthcare Assessment and Gap Analysis

- ❖ Customize any assessment to your organization needs.
- ❖ Assessments are valuable and will provide additional guidance when selecting a project.
- ❖ The assessment should be conducted on a regular basis and shared within the organization.
- ❖ When gaining consensus on scoring the various statements within the assessment, do not over-analyze. If there are different views on how a particular statement or question is phrased, make a note on how the group interpreted it, score it, and then move on. This will ensure a similar "take" of that question or statement on any subsequent assessment.

Case Study for Lean Healthcare Assessment and Gap Analysis

This clinic had recently implemented their EMR system and redesigned their lobby. However, with those changes and others, the most recent 6 month patient satisfaction scores did not improve. This had the clinic's leadership surprised and somewhat at a loss as what more to do. One of the leaders knew that Lean and Six Sigma could be used to improve the situation. A work group was formed to work with a Lean Sensei on conducting an initial assessment as well as identifying opportunities.

The assessment score indicated low values in the Process Management category, specifically areas of Process Focus, Variation, and Information being rated below average. The recommendation was: assess the patient flow through a Waste Walk, process map the flow, and identify the bottlenecks.

The data collected showed patients were waiting too long in the exam rooms to get their blood drawn. Most days, by 10:00 am, there was a backup for patients getting their blood drawn. One recommendation was to increase the number of draw stations from 1 to 4 and educate the staff to direct patients to the lab area once a request was made. This improvement made from the assessment and recommendations was used to supplement other improvements made from staff suggestions. The next 6 month survey indicated an overall increase in nearly all areas of the patient satisfaction survey. Leadership agreed to do a similar assessment every 6 months.

Stakeholder Analysis

Change the way you look at things and the things you look at change.
Wayne W. Dyer

What is it?

Stakeholder Analysis is the technique used to identify the key people who have to be influenced for a project implementation or change initiative. After analysis, stakeholder planning builds the necessary support for project success. A stakeholder is any person or organization, who can be positively or negatively impacted by, or cause an impact on the actions of a company, government, or organization. Types of stakeholders are:

Primary stakeholders: are those ultimately affected, either positively or negatively by an organization's actions.
Secondary stakeholders: are the 'intermediaries', that is, persons or organizations who are indirectly affected by an organization's actions.
Key stakeholders: (who can also belong to the first two groups) are those who control critical resources, who can block the change initiative by direct or indirect means, who must approve certain aspects of the change strategy, who shape the thinking of other critical constituents, or who own a key work process impacted by the change initiative.

What does it do?

Stakeholder Analysis is critical to the success of every project in every organization. By engaging the right people in the right way before, during, and after the completion of a major initiative (i.e., Lean Sigma or business improvement project) or change within an organization, you can make a big difference in its success.

Stakeholder Analysis develops cooperation between the stakeholders. The project team assure successful outcomes for the project. Stakeholder Analysis clarifies the consequences of proposed changes or at the start of new projects. It is important to identify all stakeholders for the purpose of identifying the stakeholder's success criteria to the project.

How do you do it?

The following steps or guidelines are used to conduct a Stakeholder Analysis:

1. Identify the stakeholders. Brainstorm who the stakeholders are in reference to the change that is about to occur or the project that is considered. List all people affected by the work, who have influence or power over it, or have an interest in its successful or unsuccessful conclusion. The following lists people who might be stakeholders in your projects:

Your boss	Shareholders	Government
Senior executives	Alliance partners	Trade associations
Your coworkers	Suppliers	The press
Your team	Lenders	Interest groups
Customers	Analysts/Consultants	The public
Prospective customers	Future employees	The community

Key questions the project manager should ask at this step are:

❖ Who is threatening the target of this project?
❖ Who is most dependent on this project?
❖ Has there been a similar project in another healthcare organization? If so, to what extent did it succeed? Who was in charge and how did local stakeholders respond?
❖ Are any government or compliance departments to be involved in this project?
❖ Are there national and/or international bodies involved in this project because of specific laws or treaties?
❖ Who are the people or groups most knowledgeable about, and capable of dealing with the project at stake?
❖ Are the stakeholders and their interests stable across the globe or are there any identifiable patterns that exist?
❖ Do major events/trends/activities currently affect the stakeholders?

2. List each stakeholder by name, title, or function along the left side of the Stakeholder Analysis and Commitment Chart. After discussion, estimate how they feel about the initiative.

For each individual, examine objective evidence (e.g., "At the last staff meeting Bill clearly stated his unwillingness to assign a member of his group to the team.") as well as subjective opinion (e.g., "Betty is likely to be strongly supportive because of her unit's objectives in this area.").

It may be useful to first have each team member rate each stakeholder without discussion, and then tally individual ratings and discuss obvious differences. While it probably is not critical to strive for complete consensus, it is usually worthwhile to take the time to generally agree on whether each key stakeholder is against, neutral, or supportive.

Before trying to come to agreement on the level of resistance, define in operational terms what "Strongly Against" means – what behaviors are seen – and also do this for the other categories. This will make consensus easier to achieve.

Stakeholder Analysis and Commitment Chart

Significance: _____

Site: _____ Desired Change _____ Date: _____
(or Project Proposal)

Names / Titles / Functions	Strongly Against (SA)	Moderately Against (MA)	Neutral (N)	Moderately Supportive (MS)	Strongly Supportive (SS)
Jim		X————————		——►O	

X = Current level of commitment
O = Minimum level of commitment to succeed
➔ = Influence links

Stakeholder Analysis

When there is general agreement each stakeholder's position, the discussion turns to where each key stakeholder needs to be for the change initiative to be successful. Remember, some stakeholders need only be shifted from Strongly Against to Neutral (meaning they will no longer be an active blocker), while others may only need to be Moderately Supportive.

Questions the project manager may ask at this step are:

- ❖ What financial or emotional interest do stakeholders have in the outcome of the project? Is it positive or negative?
- ❖ What motivates each most of all?
- ❖ What information do they want or need?
- ❖ How do they want to receive information?
- ❖ What is the best way of communicating to them?
- ❖ What is their current opinion of the project? Is it based on good information?
- ❖ Who influences their opinions generally, and who influences their opinion of this project? Do some of these influencers therefore become important stakeholders in their own right?
- ❖ If they are not likely to be positive, what will influence them to support the project?
- ❖ For those that cannot be won over, how will their opposition be managed?
- ❖ Who else might be influenced by their opinions? Do these people become stakeholders in their own right?

A very good way of answering these questions is to talk to your key stakeholders directly - people are often quite open about their views, and asking people's opinions is often the first step in building a successful relationship with them.

3. Create a Stakeholder Analysis and Resistance Chart and look for logical relationships between and among these stakeholders in terms of who might assist the team in gaining the support of others.

For example, if a key stakeholder who is Strongly Supportive is also a leader, it might be useful to enlist his/her support influencing the thinking of other less-supportive stakeholders. The more you know about the stakeholders the better prepared you are to handle their concerns regarding the project.

It is helpful to review the previously discussed resistance to change for the constituents, with regard to why key stakeholders may be against the change.

Stakeholder Analysis and Resistance Chart

Significance: _____

Site: _____ Desired Change _____ Date: _____
(or Project Proposal)

Names / Titles / Functions	SA	MA	N	MS	SS	Issues / Concerns	"Wins"	Influence Strategy

Note: This should be a confidential conversation. All assumptions are subject to validation by key stakeholders.
"Wins" - how that person can impact the project
Influence Strategy - qualities to convince or influence (direct one-on-one, charts, previous project success, etc.)

Note: Some teams use this tool to assess commitment and buy-in of individual members of the team. Though risky and probably inappropriate when a team is in the early stage of development, this can be an influential team-building exercise for a mature team. If well-facilitated and all agree to a disussion on this topic, be open and candid in their assessment and any feedback.

4. Create a Stakeholder Analysis Attitude and Influence Matrix.

This tool helps the team segment key stakeholders based upon attitude toward their project and influence to help/block results. The matrix provides a visual, political map. It answers the questions: *Who are the stakeholders? Where do they currently stand on the issues associated with this change initiative? What is their attitude?* and *How much Influence do they possess to enable or disable?* This tool assumes that: 1) a critical mass is essential for launching/accelerating the change effort and identifies where the greatest concentration of support exists, 2) some stakeholders can be moved to a higher level of support, and 3) high influence constituencies are important and can impact project success.

This tool can be used when the team is ready for a discussion of specific individuals and how these stakeholders currently view the change initiative. It can also be used throughout the process to strategize about how to influence a new stakeholder who may have just emerged.

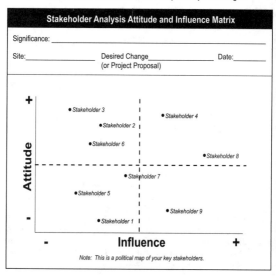

5. Identify key stakeholders who provide a positive attitude to other key stakeholders.

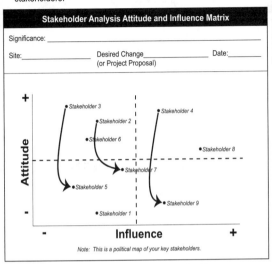

Stakeholder Analysis Attitude and Influence Matrix

Significance: _____

Site: _____ Desired Change _____ Date: _____
(or Project Proposal)

Note: This is a political map of your key stakeholders.

Step 6. Create and implement a Stakeholder Action Plan.

The Stakeholder Action Plan is a variant of the WWWW - Who (does), What (by), When, and Why - common in project management techniques. Once key stakeholders are known and their attitudes have been discussed (and validated through private one-on-one meetings), team efforts turn to building an effective strategy for influencing them to strengthen, or at a minimum, maintain their level of support. The team's task is to determine what actions need to be taken to influence the stakeholder in question, who can best influence each individual listed that requires influencing, and when specific actions will be taken. This tool is very straightforward and easy to understand. Careful thought needs to be given about who will have most impact on any particular individual, what will be done to influence them, and when should the influence process begin.

When the team has validated their understanding of the stakeholders' issues and concerns, it is time to proceed with developing an influence strategy. At this point, it is often useful to consider the following aspects of the influence process which may not have been addressed before:

❖ What is this person's style? E.g., Is he/she a numbers person who will be swayed by data and statistics?
❖ What history needs to be taken into account as we talk with this individual? Has he/she been negatively impacted by similar initiatives in the past? Does he/she have an issue with any of the team members that might make it difficult to support the initiative?
❖ Is there a part of the change initiative that we can give them ownership to secure their support?

Ensure the influence strategy will be implemented appropriately and in a timely fashion.

Stakeholder Action Plan				
Significance:				
Site:	Desired Change (or Project Proposal)			Date:
Stakeholder	What	Who	When	Why

The following benefits can be obtained by conducting a Stakeholder Analysis:

❖ Opinions of the most powerful stakeholders are revealed at an early stage
❖ Support from powerful stakeholders will help obtain adequate resources - making it more likely that the projects will be successful
❖ Communication with stakeholders early and frequently will help ensure that everyone fully understands what the project is about and its benefits
❖ Anticipation of people's reaction to the project may win them over early

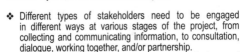

Sensei Tips for Stakeholder Analysis

- ❖ Different types of stakeholders need to be engaged in different ways at various stages of the project, from collecting and communicating information, to consultation, dialogue, working together, and/or partnership.
- ❖ Determining who needs or wants to be involved, and when and how that involvement can be achieved provides the basis for acceptance.
- ❖ Once stakeholder views are understood, a decision can be made on whether to pursue collaboration and the types of communication that will be required before, during, and after the project.
- ❖ The Stakeholder Analysis tool should be used with strict confidentiality.
- ❖ Experience shows that successful, sustained change is difficult to achieve without attention from the entire team.
- ❖ Every change initiative will compete for time, resources, and attention.
- ❖ We often spend most available time on the launch of an initiative rather than its institutionalization (or in Lean terms, standardization of change).
- ❖ Create consistent and visible reinforcement of the change initiative.
- ❖ Integrate the new initiative with ongoing work patterns.
- ❖ Identify changes to organizational systems and structures that help make the change a natural part of individual and team behavior.

Case Study for Stakeholder Analysis

In this Physician Group Practice, the Office Manager, Judy, had worked with an outside consultant, two X-ray techs, and one physician. Dr. Quinn was willing to change to increase throughput for new patients and eliminate the number of returning patients that were being rescheduled. Patients were rescheduled due to not having the proper X-ray views when the doctors were meeting with the patient. The doctor's perception was that the X-ray techs were underutilized and did not understand why they were constantly working overtime as well as behind schedule throughout the day.

On a side note, Dr. Hahn, and a few other doctors, vocalized their displeasure with the implementation of the new EMR system; it appeared to create more work for them and their PAs. Many of the doctors liked the things the way there were and did not like change.

The team proposed a revised protocol for the "standard" number of views for the top 5 body areas (knee, shoulder, etc.) for returning patients. For example, the new protocol required that a returning patient left knee would receive 5 shots (views).

The team discussed how to ensure a successful roll-out of this new protocol. The consultant conveyed that the roll-out will likely have various degrees of resistance, and therefore, the communication of the proposed change, will be different depending on the doctor.

Dr. Martinez was working part-time, only seeing 10 patients per day. On the other hand, Dr. Hahn was seeing nearly 50 patients a day and additional efforts in terms of one-on-one meetings, asking for his feedback in the beginning and throughout the implementation, as well as sharing the proposed productivity (ROI) numbers, helped him with accepting the change. Another activity was to have two "lunch-and-learns" to help communicate the need for change as well as entertain questions.

The consultant recommended a Stakeholder Analysis be conducted.

The Stakeholder Analysis results are shown below:

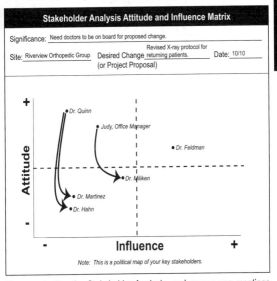

Stakeholder Analysis Attitude and Influence Matrix

Significance: Need doctors to be on board for proposed change.

Site: Riverview Orthopedic Group   Desired Change: Revised X-ray protocol for returning patients.   Date: 10/10
(or Project Proposal)

Note: This is a political map of your key stakeholders.

From conducting the Stakeholder Analysis, and one-on-one meetings with each physician to confirm their current attitude regarding this desired change, it was determined that Dr. Quinn would approach both Drs. Martinez and Hahn and solicit their support (as well as address any concerns). Judy, the Office Manager, had a good relationship with Dr. Miliken and felt she could also work with him.

After 30 days with the new protocol, the number of returning patients needed to be rescheduled due to not having the correct views was reduced by 43%. Also, it reduced the number of same day patients of not having to go back and get additional views taken by 33%, which also impacted the patient's length of visit. With the changes being done in this manner, there was an increase of patients seen by 10%.

Dr. Hahn was so impressed with the results, he requested that the team look at their scheduling system, and he would be more than happy to participate any way he could!

Project Identification

It's not that I'm so smart, it's just that I stay with problems longer.
Albert Einstein

What is it?

Project Identification is the process of determining areas that are not meeting performance or operational goals. Determining the project requires data from Balanced Scorecards, Performance Dashboards, Voice of the Customer surveys, competitor's product or service, market demands, customer/patient surveys, etc.

What does it do?

The Balanced Scorecard, Performance Dashboard, etc. may help identify major areas (i.e., value streams) where improvement efforts will need to be focused. However, there may be times where the management group (or continuous improvement group) requires additional guidelines to select the appropriate project to obtain the most bang-for-your-buck. In these cases it may be helpful to create a Project Prioritization Worksheet and/or Distribution Report.

The **Project Prioritization Worksheet** is a listing of the main areas of concern relative to the significant factors important to the organization.

The **Distribution Report** is a historical listing on the volume of work or service completed within a specific time period for a department or work group.

Using the Project Prioritization Worksheet and/or Distribution Report will help to assure the resources are being committed in a responsible manner.

How do you do it?

The following steps or guidelines are used to create and use a Project Prioritization Worksheet and/or Distribution Report:

1. Identify area(s) throughout the organization that need improvement (from the Balanced Scorecard, Voice of the Customer surveys, value streams analysis, etc.).

2. Create a Project Prioritization Worksheet by following these steps:

   a. List all (1) Areas/Processes that require immediate improvement.
   b. Place a check mark in each Area/Process applicable to the category of (2) Impacts Customer or Patient, (3) Affects Safety, (4) High Volume, (5) Over Budget, (6) Demand Exceeds Capacity, (7) Customer or Patient Dissatisfier, (8) Supplier Dissatisfier, (9) Staff Dissatisfier, and (10) Never Goes Right. These may have multiple selections. Select the top three-to-five.
   c. Tally the points for each row (11) Total Points. Use the data to select core team members for the identified project.

(1) Areas/Processes	(2) Impacts Customer or Patient	(3) Affects Safety	(4) High Volume	(5) Over Budget	(6) Demand Exceeds Capacity	(7) Customer or Patient Dissatisfier	(8) Supplier Dissatisfier	(9) Staff Dissatisfier	(10) Never Goes Right	(11) Total Points
Pt Arrival	✔	✔			✔	✔		✔		5
Registration								✔		1
Triage			✔	✔	✔			✔		4
Bed Assign								✔	✔	2
Ns Assess		✔		✔		✔				3
Phys Assess	✔	✔			✔					3
Lab		✔				✔		✔	✔	4
Radiology		✔				✔		✔	✔	4
Other Anc						✔		✔	✔	3
Pharmacy		✔						✔	✔	3
Disposition	✔	✔	✔		✔	✔	✔			6
Instructions		✔	✔		✔	✔		✔		5
Discharge	✔	✔	✔	✔	✔	✔	✔		✔	8

Project Identification

3. Create a Distribution Report (examples shown below) by following these steps:

   a. Determine data collection method (i.e., database retrieval, direct observation, Voice of the Customer, etc.).
   b. Organize the data by volume and other key attributes for the data set.
   c. Present the data in a report or chart.

Department (reasons why pts come to the hospital)	Pts/month	Registration	OP Scheduling	Transport	Housekeeping	Medical Records
IP visit/surgery	457	X		X	X	X
OP Surgery	140	X	X	X	X	X
OP Laboratory	230	X				X
OP Radiology	160	X	X		X	X
Clinic visit	178	X	X		X	X
ED visit	2950	X		X	X	X
Pharmacy visit	124					X
OP Phys/Occ Therapy	85	X	X		X	X
Community classes	425				X	X

Time Periods	March 1	March 2	March 3	March 4	March 6	March 7	March 8	March 10	March 11	March 12	March 13	March 14	March 15	Totals	Average Volume Volume Per 4 Hours
0000 - 0400	4	3	2	5	4	4	4	3	2	4	5	4	5	5	6	60	4
0400 - 0800	7	7	8	12	10	7	9	9	10	12	9	8	8	10	9	135	9
0800 - 1200	14	15	20	15	17	18	16	20	18	17	20	15	14	17	19	255	17
1200 - 1600	18	22	28	27	28	29	30	28	27	26	27	28	30	22	20	390	26
1600 - 2000	40	32	35	32	30	28	26	35	38	31	33	28	30	28	34	480	32
2000 - 2400	14	18	18	16	19	16	14	17	14	17	18	15	18	20	21	255	17
													TOTAL		1575	

4. Use the data to create the Team or Project Charter (see Define Phase) and/or A3 Reports (next section).

The following benefits can be obtained by using Project Identification:

   ❖ Ensure resources are being committed in the designated areas
   ❖ Allow managers an avenue for discussions regarding potential improvement projects
   ❖ Provide the appropriate data to select the project

Sensei Tips for Project Identification

❖ The more clearly defined the projects are from the beginning, the more likelihood for success.
❖ Healthcare is traditionally data rich but information poor. Lean thinking allows you to turn data into great information.
❖ Microsoft Excel has numerous chart options to present and turn the data into useful information (very helpful while defining the project).
❖ Make sincere efforts to gain a consensus when selecting the project. Create the appropriate "What's-In-It-For-Me?" statements for staff.
❖ Use with Balanced Scorecards, value stream maps, etc. to help select (or prioritize) improvement projects.
❖ Allows for a project team to review all main processes.
❖ It can provide the framework for an initial value stream map.
❖ Helps teams "see" the big picture on how processes are connected.

Case Study for Project Identification

This multi-specialty clinic was recently purchased by a large healthcare system that has over 15 hospitals in their group. The clinic had always been profitable; however, over the past year their patient satisfaction scores have been stagnant. The new system required the clinic to report on their continuous improvement efforts on a monthly basis. Patient satisfaction was one of the many other key areas.

A Continuous Improvement Specialist (CIS) from the system was assigned to work with the clinic. A later determination would be made if it warranted that to be a full time position. The CIS met with the board to determine a good first project. The board and the CIS spent less than 30 minutes and the following is their Project Prioritization Worksheet.

(1) Services	Categories										(11) Total Points
	(2) Impacts Customer or Patient	(3) Affects Safety	(4) High Volume	(5) Over Budget	(6) Demand Exceeds Capacity	(7) Customer or Patient Dissatisfier	(8) Opportunity for Growth	(9) Staff Dissatisfier	(10) Never Goes Right		
Cardiology	✔	✔		✔	✔	✔	✔	✔			8
Family Practice					✔			✔			2
Endocrinology	✔				✔	✔	✔	✔			5
Imaging Services			✔					✔	✔		3
Pediatrics		✔					✔				2
Podiatry	✔		✔		✔	✔			✔		5

The Project Prioritization Worksheet listed Cardiology as the project selected; however, the CIS suggested more data be used in determining their first project. The following is a Data Distribution Report. The "X" indicates a link between the patient satisfaction survey and the various services.

Service Lines	Pts/month Projected	Pts/month Actual	Registration	Scheduling	Patient Care Giver Engagement	Cleanliness	Billing
Cardiology	400	428	X				X
Family Practice	760	866		X	X	X	X
Endocrinology	266	230	X	X	X	X	X
Imaging Services	238	220	X	X		X	X
Pediatrics	638	644		X	X	X	X
Podiatry	78	82				X	X

These two reports, along with the financial reporting of Endo not meeting their projection of 266 patients per month, clearly identified the focus (i.e., value stream). This also provided the best ROI on resource allocations for the first project. The board was impressed with this initial assessment and was in full support of the efforts moving forward. Often more than one information source will be used to identify a project.

A3 Reports

A vision without a plan is just a dream.
A plan without a vision is just drudgery.
But a vision with a plan can change the world!

Unknown

What is it?

The **A3 Report** is designed to help you "tell the story" in a logical and visual way with reference to a particular subject matter. The A3 refers to size 11" X 17" paper, however, in today's applications it can be any type of medium that is easily viewed. The main types of A3 Reports are: Continuous Improvement and Problem Solving (or Project) - the focus of this section, Status, Proposal, and Strategic (or Hoshin) Planning. The A3 Project Report was originally developed by Toyota to represent a problem or improvement initiative in the field with paper.

There are typically eight categories of an A3 Project Report; however, there may be more or less depending on the project. For example, step 7. Verify Results (next page) may be divided into Pre-Metrics and Post-Metrics, or, step 1. Problem Statement may be renamed to Current Business Case, etc. The overall purpose for this tool is to efficiently display relevant information on one sheet of paper (or Desktop/Tablet page or screen) in a logical sequence as well as be a reporting or tool application road map for your project. Relevant data or information should be represented on the A3, however if the information does not fit, additional sheets may be used and referenced on the A3 Report.

What does it do?

The A3 Report provides a consistent approach for learning, applying, and documenting Lean Six Sigma tools used. It is simple and typically organized as a series of boxes in a template. The A3 Report will help employees "think" Lean.

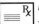

How do you do it?

The following are the main A3 Project Report sections:

Note: The A3 Report can be created in Excel or a similar program, sized and printed on size A3 paper (or smaller).

1. Problem Statement - Define the business problem, issue, or specific improvement project.

2. Current State - Describe the current state by completing a process or value stream map, a graph or chart denoting a negative trend, etc.

3. Improvement Opportunity - Identify the desired outcomes and targets.

4. Problem Analysis - Examine the process in detail using a Fishbone Diagram, Brainstorming, 5 Why Analysis, Impact Map, etc.

5. Future State - Create a future state free of waste.

6. Implementation Plan - List the specific steps, Who, What, When, etc. for the process changes (referred to as PDCAs) and complete.

7. Verify Results - Show before and after measurements using good charting methods.

8. Follow-Up - Create a plan for system-wide roll-out, if applicable, training, and possibly use SPC and Visual Management principles to monitor and sustain process changes.

The following aligns the D-M-A-I-C Phases with the eight main categories of the A3 Project Report:

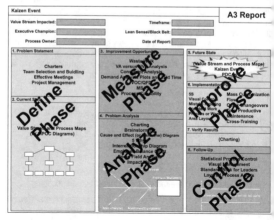

The following questions will ensure the Problem Statement section is complete prior to moving on the next section of the A3 Project Report. (The entire list of questions for each part of the A3 Project Report is contained in the Appendix, pages 232 - 234.)

Define Phase

1. Problem Statement

What data do we have to support the significance of the problem?
What percent of the time are we meeting patient/customer expectations?
What is the impact of the problem on the customers of the process?
What is the "Business Line of Sight" between our strategic goals and dashboards, to this particular issue?

Note: There is an Add-On for MS Office Excel called QI Macros that has over 90 charts and graphs for assisting in data presentation and analysis. It is a fill-in-the-blanks for chart and documentation templates (the A3 being one of them). Also, check the iTunes stores for the Practical Lean Six Sigma for Healthcare Series - A3 Report app.

The following benefits can be obtained by using the A3 Report:

- ❖ Provide a single, easy-to-use approach for any type of problem solving or continuous improvement project
- ❖ Free people up to focus on the root causes of problems - without needing to reinvent new ways of reporting
- ❖ Stimulate dialogue and creative problem solving, and build consensus based on objective facts
- ❖ Break people of the bad habit of jumping to solutions
- ❖ Instill an organizational culture of "learning to learn"
- ❖ Groom new leaders to solve problems in a scientifically repeatable (i.e., standard) way
- ❖ Provide a systematic logical thinking process
- ❖ Teach people to identify a problem or opportunity, understand and "see" cause and effect relationships at-a-glance
- ❖ Be used along with any improvement methodology

Note: The A3 Project Reports under Sensei Tips are reduced images and the text details are not the focus. Each A3 is noted at the bottom of the image for its uniqueness. A larger image of these can be obtained by requesting the page number to info@ theleanstore.com. *The A3 Pocket Handbook for Kaizen Events* is a good book for team members to reference, follow-along, and document individual and team activities of a Kaizen Event.

The following are examples of A3 Project Reports:

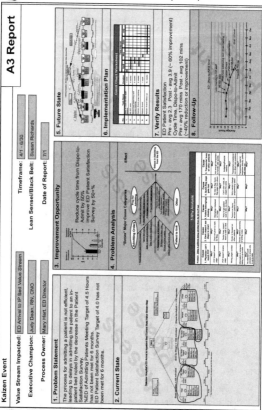

This A3 Project Report conveys some of the main Lean tools (i.e., value stream maps, Fishbone Diagram, Pareto Chart, Gantt Chart, etc.) used in this ED improvement team project.

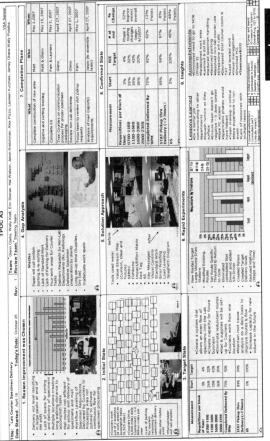

Note the use of actual photos in "telling the story" for this hospital lab example as well as their customized nine categories.

Prepare

ED RADIOLOGY TAT

Process Owner: Jan Hopkins and Joe Myers	Executive Sponsor: Connie Franklin

Facilitator / Co-Facilitator: Jennifer Carter, Greg Booth, Stacy Cupid, Michelle Marrow, Deanne Troy

Measurements	Start	% Improvement	Day 1	Day 2	Day 3	Day 4	Target
Order Entry to Exam Start (Minutes)	35 (n=1700)	23%	17 (n=70)	31 (n=70)	12 (n=58)	27 (n=9)	25
Yield	55%	To be measured 1 week after start of new process (July 27)					80%
Percent Orders Correct	86%	To be measured 1 week after start of new process (July 27)					100%
Top Box	44%	To be measured 2 months after of new process (September)					50%

Major Accomplishments

- **Developed ED Radiology communication record**
- Streamlined patient transport to X-Ray
- Utilized FirstNet tracking board for communication
- Improved patient safety
- Improved X-Ray documentation
- Improved patient readiness
- Created a PULL system
- Created a visual cue for RNs and physicians
- Decreased number of phone calls
- Allowed the nurse to stay at bedside
- Allowed Rad Tech to stay within department
- Educated physicians on unnecessary tests
- Improved communication between departments

Eliminated 9 Non Value-Added Steps

Streamlined 13 Steps

Future State

Standard Kaizen Week:
July 16-20

Note the good sample size used in the data collection phase (i.e., n=1700).

Providence, Non-Invasive Cardiology

Process Owner: Julie O'Mallery | Project Sponsor: Kathy Smith

Facilitator / Co-Facilitator: Kate Blanchart, Mike Eisle, Greg Both, Sue Lanwodowski

Metrics	"Before"	Target	"After"	% Improved
CT: Stress Echo	12 hours	6 hours	8 hours	33%
CT: Resting Echo	12 hours	6 hours	8 hours	33%
CT: Stress Nuclear	18 hours	9 hours	9 hours	50%
# Carryover	3 / 15	0 / 0 / 0	0 / 0 / 0	100%

Major Accomplishments:

- Improved/clarified placement of stress test on chest pain pathway
- Improved flow with additional Transporter assignment
- Decreased unnecessary motion and transportation
- Developed visual cue for "Patient NPO" prior to test
- Implemented sharing of testing schedule throughout nursing units
- Improved Cardiologist rounding to read exams more quickly
- Developed visual cues for stat and urgent interpretations by Cardiologists
- Estimated savings: $92,000

RIE Week:
February 6

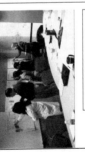

Note the involvement of all the team members while they created the current state value stream map as shown in the lower left portion of this A3 Project Report.

A3 Reports

Lean Thinking Statements for Prepare

The following Lean Thinking Statement assessment should be done as an individual and, if desired, combined and discussed as a team. If the team leader realizes that many of the items are an issue for certain team members, then maybe a one-on-one with those specific individuals would be appropriate. Or, if a few of the team members have similar concerns over one or two of the statements, then possibly these should be addressed with the team. Open honest dialogue with the team at the beginning of the project ensures a good start. As a team member, it is YOUR responsibility to address any of the statements that hinder YOUR individual input to the team's progress. These statements are not to be taken lightly!

Use the 5 Level Likert Scale for the following statements:

> 1 - Strongly Disagree
> 2 - Disagree
> 3 - Neither Agree nor Disagree
> 4 - Agree
> 5 - Strongly Agree

I am aware that current measurements are not acceptable. ———
I understand the need for change. ———
I believe resources will be made available for this project. ———
I believe the process owner is onboard. ———
I am confident that upper management will support the improvements proposed by the team. ———
I believe all stakeholders will eventually support our efforts. ———
I am confident in discussing this project with my colleagues. ———
I see the value in this team's approach. ———
I believe I can add value to this team. ———
I believe my ideas will be heard and considered. ———

Total Score: [   ]

If your score is less than 80% (40 points), then more preparation should be completed before moving on to the Define Phase. Ensure that an A3 Project Report or similar tool has been created that can then be used throughout the scope of the project.

The Define Phase

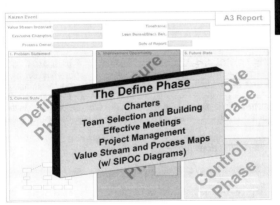

The Define Phase

Charters
Team Selection and Building
Effective Meetings
Project Management
Value Stream and Process Maps
(w/ SIPOC Diagrams)

Tools listed in this section are most likely to be used at this time.
All the tools can be applicable at any phase of a Kaizen Project as
determined by the needs of the project team.

Charters

Good management is the art of making problems so interesting and their solutions so constructive that everyone wants to go to work and deal with them.

Paul Hawken

What is it?

There are two types of Charters: the Project Charter and the Team Charter. *The **Project Charter** is a high level document used to launch or initiate improvement teams.* It is usually initiated by leadership and targeted at a major improvement need of the organization.

*The **Team Charter** documents the team structure, membership, and overall objectives, measures, and resources required for an improvement project to be successful.* It is developed by the project team and is used to fully explore the scope and resources required to complete an improvement project. Multiple Team Charters may be derived from the Project Charter, or simply, a Project Charter can be modified to be the Team Charter.

What does it do?

The purpose of Charters are to:

❖ Document reasons for the project
❖ Provide objectives and constraints of the project (prevent scope creep)
❖ Provide directions about the solution
❖ Identify main stakeholders
❖ Identify overall goals or performance expectations

Team and Project Charters define the overall scope of how and why resources of the organization are being committed to an area or process. Charters contain varying degrees of information. Charters should be communicated to the appropriate employees and updated as changes occur.

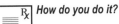

How do you do it?

The following steps or guidelines are used to create a Team Charter: (Similar steps are used to create the Project Charter; however, we are only presenting the more common Team Charter steps.)

1. Use information from the Project Charter, value stream or process map, Performance Dashboard, etc. to obtain the appropriate measurements.

2. Ensure the specific project team has had input into the development of the Team Charter.

3. Submit the Team Charter to the Team Champion or Sponsor (i.e., the person who can commit the resources) for approval.

4. Customize the Team Charter for any internal or external issues the organization may be facing.

5. Post or publish the Team Charter so it is available for everyone to view.

6. Refer back to the Team Charter if the team is struggling with direction or focus.

7. Update the Team Charter as changes occur.

The following benefits can be obtained by using a Team Charter:

❖ Ensure teams will stay on-task and not attempt to do more than what is required
❖ Ensure alignment between management and organizational improvements
❖ Encourage communication at all levels
❖ Reduce project related stress on team members

Sensei Tips for Charters

❖ Charters provides a standard format for the allocation and prioritization of resources in an organization; projects can be ranked and authorized by Return on Investment (ROI), quality improvements, patient safety, improvement of patient throughput, departmental improvements, etc.

❖ Charters serve as the primary sales document for the project ensuring the project receives the appropriate priority.

❖ Team Charters are separate, distinct, and manageable projects to be undertaken by various teams within an organization.

Case Study for Charters

The Project Charter on this page (circled portion of Team Projects) was used to create the Team Charter on the following page.

Project Charter

Mission

We will achieve success when we are able to provide efficient, clinically-effective care in a way that meets - and exceeds - our patients' needs. Clinical quality will be the foundation of our success as we strive to maintain a reasonable operating margin.

Value Statement

The process of admitting a patient has two goals; efficiency in the process and patient in the right bed the first time. Patients need to be moved from the ED as quickly as possible meeting the needs of the patient and families.

Deliverables

1. Create Operational Excellence Teams in all departments.
2. Conduct separate monthly Balanced Scorecard meetings to view progress on negative trends.
3. Support all continuous improvement teams with leadership present at all "kick-off" improvement team meetings.
4. Ensure Executive Sponsors are part of all improvement teams.

Strategic Goals

In support of the strategic goals, we will continue to focus our efforts to improve our goals as they should align with departmental goals.

Finance Goals

Operating Margin %	4.0
Adj Cost per Equiv Admit	7500

Quality Goals

Bundles, % of 100%	100
Mortality Rate, Var from Norm	< -1.0
Falls per 100 Pt Days	< 2.5

Service (Cycle Time) Goals

ED % of Admitted Patients Meeting Target (4.5 hrs)	85
OR % On-time Case Starts	85
LOS, Med-Surg (Days)	3.5

Satisfaction Goals

Inpatient Satisfaction	4.0
ED Satisfaction	4.0
OR Satisfaction	4.0
Physician Satisfaction	4.0
Employee Satisfaction	4.0

Team Projects

Emergency Department
Reduce ED LOS for Dispo-to-Admit
Reduce ED LOS for Admit Patients
Improve ED (Patient) Satisfaction scores

Surgical Services/OR
Improve OR % On-time Case Starts
Improve LOS, Med-Surg Days
Improve OR (Patient) Satisfaction scores

Outpatient and Clinical Support
Improve Physician Satisfaction scores
Complete EMR/EMS roll-out

Expected Results

Benefits (What results will be gained?)	Metrics (How will the results be measured?)
1. Improvement in all Balanced Scorecard metrics. 2. Increased knowledge of continuous improvement tools and methods. 3. Increased involvement by all employees to improving patient and non-patient care processes.	1. Departmental metrics aligned to Balanced Scorecard metrics. 2. All improvement teams to report out to management at pre-determined times for any and all Kaizen Events.

Team Charter

Team Name
ED Improvement Team

Team Members
Mary, JoAnn, Dave, Judy, John, Susan, Beth, Robert (Exec. Champion)

Outcomes
The team will create a streamlined process flow to achieve the following:
Reduce ED LOS for Dispo-to-Admit approx. 50% (from 170 mins to 90 mins)
Reduce ED LOS for Admit Patients by 25% (from 360 mins to 270 mins)
Improve ED (Patient) Satisfaction score by 50%

Deliverables
1. Create a current and future state value stream map of the ED patient experience.
2. Create and implement new standard work for the process of Dispo-to-Admit.
3. Create a Failure Prevention Analysis Worksheet to ensure mistake proofing of any process change.
4. Train all staff on new standards. Implement a 5S program throughout the ED.
5. Monitor changes (and adjust if necessary) to ensure changes are controlled and sustained over time.

Expected Scope/Approach/Activities
1. The scope of the team's authority and focus is: ED processes between physician order to admit and patient being placed into the bed. Changes to be approved during the event by the Process Owner, ED Manager, and Bed Placement Coordinator, with communication/training for other stakeholders as appropriate.
2. In addition to the week-long focused Kaizen Event, the team will conduct preparatory meetings as needed to support the Event week, including contacting IT and facilities for expected support during the Event week.

Strategic Alignment Factors
- ED LOS for Admitted Patients
- Efficiency (decreased time in the ED places pt more quickly in less costly care on the inpatient unit)
- Growth (opening capacity and decreasing "Left Without Being Seen" for other patients)
- Clinical Effectiveness (care by the ED physician is focused on immediate conditions, while care by the admitting physician is focused on the patient's short and long term needs)

Team Process

Process Item	Frequency	Audience/Distribution
Stakeholder Check	• Daily, during, and 30-60-90 day post-Event	• Team members, face-to-face, for all stakeholders
Information Distribution	• Once, after first preparatory meetings • Daily, after each day of the Event • 30-60-90 day follow-up	• From team to stakeholders, after first preparatory meeting • From team to entire hospital staff
Team Meetings	• Three prep meetings in three weeks prior • Daily, during the Event, weekly follow-ups	• Team, Process Owner, Champion • Team, Process Owner, Facilitator
Status Reporting	• 30-60-90 Follow-up reports	• Team, Process Owner, Fac., Champion

Expected Results

Benefits (What results will be gained?)	Metrics (How will the results be measured?)
1. Reduced cycle time, Dispo-to-Admit by approx. 50% 2. Improved ED Patient Satisfaction by 50+%	1. Cycle time metrics collected weekly 2. Patient Satisfaction scores, weekly mean scores

Assumptions
- ED patient volumes will remain consistent
- ED staffing will support change

Risks
- ED staff will not follow new standards
- Some stakeholders will not support change

Internal Issues
- ED physicians not engaged after admit order written
- Disagreement among physicians who should write order
- Staffing concerns with nursing
- Nurse Planning may relieve staff on units due to low census

External Issues
- Joint Commission's new requirements on patient hand-offs and transportation between units

This Team Charter is created out of the previous Project Charter Team Projects section - Emergency Department. It includes all the information for an improvement team to get started as well as provide specific direction.

Define

Team Selection and Building

On this team, we're all united in a common goal: to keep my job.
Lou Holtz

What is it?

Team selection is the process of selecting people to work together on a team. **Team building** is the process of leading a group of people on a team in a way that strengthens bonds and cohesiveness in order to achieve harmony and success. Teaming can be done in-person (i.e., face-to-face) or through the use of remote communications via Web-collaboration applications or tools. The principles of teaming are the same regardless of the industry, type of project, or communication platform.

What does it do?

The prospect of collaborating with your co-workers, e.g., physicians, nurses, techs, transporters, admin, etc. can be frightening for many leaders because they have been trained in management where they should know the answers. Building an effective team and enabling them to solve problems through teaming may be foreign to many healthcare leaders.

How do you do it?

There are many methods of team selection. Diversity may be achieved through cross-functional teams, personality assessments, or unique skill assessments. Whichever methods are used, leaders must strive for a diversified, yet balanced, team make-up. Use the following steps or guidelines (also referred to as the five stages of teaming) to select and lead a team:

1. Form the team. The **Forming** stage (or step) of teaming involves reviewing the project, establishing team roles, determining meeting times, and ensuring the right members are on the team. There is excitement, anticipation, and optimism. There is also the pride a member feels since he or she has been chosen to be part of the team. The "flip-side" are feelings of suspicion, fear, and anxiety about what is to come.

2. Facilitate the team through their ***Storming*** stage. At this stage, the team members begin to realize the task is different and/or more difficult than they first imagined. This is the stage where the team members experience difficulties transitioning from working as individuals to contributing as a team member. Impatience about the lack of progress and inexperience on group dynamics has some team members wondering about the entire project. This stage can be difficult for any team. Teams that do not understand and acknowledge the five stages - especially this stage - most likely will disband or experience sub-par performance.

3. Monitor and reward as progress is being made. This stage is referred to as the ***Norming*** stage. Team members accept the team concept. At this stage, the team ground rules are adhered to, communication is occurring without disruptions, progress is being made toward the objective, and everyone feels that the team concept is working. Everyone is contributing in a positive way. Continued communications and acknowledgement of the team members' efforts should be done often, allowing progress to Stage 4 and preventing the team from falling back to Stage 2.

4. Effectively solve problems and involve everyone on the team. By the time this ***Performing*** stage has been reached, the team can begin to diagnose and solve problems with relative ease. Every member is contributing and time is being leveraged to its fullest. Team members may be selected to assist other teams, start new projects, etc.

5. Learn and share results. Closure of the project team is the final stage of teaming. In this ***Closing*** stage, the team has accomplished their goals, shared their results, and has disbanded. Closure brings mixed feelings to team members. By this time, the team members have been through a lot together and the thought of not working as a team anymore can be disappointing. However, project teams are not usually designed to be together forever. An organization's structure handles the long-term team structure. Improvement teams are, by nature, cross-functional and have a specific purpose and life.

The following benefits can be obtained for proper team selection and building:

❖ Engage the employees
❖ Create a 'willingness to share' culture
❖ Allow for better decision-making
❖ Encourage diversity of ideas

Sensei Tips for Team Selection and Building

The following are examples of teams at various stages:

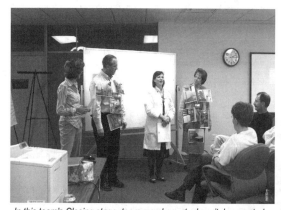

In this team's Closing stage, team members at a hospital presented a "live" storyboard of their improvement project to the department.

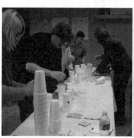

This team's Forming stage included training for their Lean Sigma project via a simulation to help staff to understand Lean Six Sigma concepts.

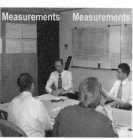

This team's Storming stage meetings were held in the conference room. The measurements are posted to keep the team focused on the objectives.

Case Study for Team Selection and Building

Linda, a newly hired office manager for a 19-cardiologist group practice, was immediately challenged to improve overall patient satisfaction scores. The recent survey addressed the following areas: access (ease of getting through on the phone, ease of getting an appointment, waiting times); communication between patient and office (quality of health information materials, ability to get a call returned, getting tests results back quickly); staff (courtesy of the receptionist, caring of nurses and medical assistants, helpfulness of people in the business office); and the interaction with the doctors (whether the doctor listens, thoroughness of explanations and instructions, whether the doctors take time to answer questions, how much time the doctors spend with the patient). The areas that showed a significant decline from the survey conducted six months prior were waiting times and how much time the doctors spend with the patient.

Linda decided to create two teams and she was to be the Team Co-Champion, along with Dr. Ellis, the CEO of the practice. Linda posted the survey results in the break room, and sent a copy to their email addresses. Linda announced that two teams were to be formed and if someone had an interest to let her know. Linda wanted 5 staff per team. Within a week, and a little more communication from Linda, she had the volunteers.

Linda held the first meeting with both teams and conducted a short training session on process/continuous improvement, as well as reviewed and discussed the five stages of team development. Linda had informed both groups of the structured methodology of D-M-A-I-C that will keep the team focused and on track. Linda held the meetings on Tuesdays and Thursdays from 12 – 1 and provided lunch. She wanted both teams to not look at this as an arduous task, but a time when and where improvement ideas can be explored and discussed prior to any changes, thus creating a positive experience for everyone.

There was little argument from the team members, as Linda kept the team meetings short and to-the-point. To demonstrate continuous improvement for the teaming process, and to respect everyone's time and commitment to it, Linda distributed the following Team Survey (next page) at various stages throughout the project and subsequently addressed each main issue.

Team Survey

Directions:

1. Read each statement carefully.
2. Use the 5-level Likert Item scale.
3. Circle the response that best expresses your feelings about that statement.

Rating System: Use the following 5-level Likert Item scale:

1 - Strongly Disagree
2 - Disagree
3 - Neither Agree nor Disagree
4 - Agree
5 - Strongly Agree

	Strongly Disagree	Disagree	Neither Agree nor Disagree	Agree	Strongly Agree
1. My team has clearly defined the goals and purpose for our being together as a team.	1	2	3	4	5
2. My team practices mutual support and backup on the topics that we discussed at the meeting.	1	2	3	4	5
3. My team communicates well which includes having an agenda before the meeting and providing action items within 24 hours after.	1	2	3	4	5
4. My team practices constructive criticism.	1	2	3	4	5
5. My team has trust in one another.	1	2	3	4	5
6. My team has clearly defined roles and responsibilities.	1	2	3	4	5
7. My team has diverse skills, knowledge, and abilities.	1	2	3	4	5
8. My team has clear rules or standards when we meet.	1	2	3	4	5
9. Team rules are enforced in a firm but fair manner.	1	2	3	4	5
10. My team is self-disciplined and motivated to accomplish its goals.	1	2	3	4	5
11. My team leader effectively manages our meeting times.	1	2	3	4	5
12. My team leader has made him/herself available after meetings.	1	2	3	4	5
13. My team leader is motivated to lead this team.	1	2	3	4	5
14. My team will be successful.					
15. My team has all the resources required to accomplish its goals.	1	2	3	4	5
16. All actions items were assigned equitably.	1	2	3	4	5
17. The results of this survey will be used honestly and constructively by this team to improve my teaming experience.	1	2	3	4	5

Please include any other ideas/comments that you feel would improve this team's experience:

_____

_____

_____

Do not sign your name. All responses will be kept in strict confidence.

Within 4 weeks, the team had some recommendations for the Improve Phase. The main recommendation was to request patients to arrive only 15 minutes ahead of schedule, versus the current 30 minutes. It was also suggested that 10% of the cardiologists pay be based on a combination of patient and peer satisfaction surveys.

The team presented the recommendations to Dr. Ellis with additional information collected throughout the Measure and Analyze Phases. Dr. Ellis was impressed with the detail (i.e., useful data) that suggested these improvements would improve the overall patient satisfaction survey. Dr. Ellis subsequently agreed to the 10% compensation plan (after meeting and explaining this to the other partners and cardiologists).

Linda and the team monitored the improvements in the Control Phase. Linda rewarded each team member with a $50.00 gift card. At the next survey, both areas had improved significantly.

Effective Meetings

When you go to meetings or auditions and you fail to prepare, prepare to fail. It is that simple.
Paula Abdul

What is it?

An **effective meeting** is an efficient use of people's time when they are gathered together working to obtain a desired result. Meetings, like any process, can be studied and improved upon. Meetings can be one of the most powerful business tools. While many decisions can be made by phone, email, or in hallway discussions, there will be other times that people will need to meet (in person or through Web conferencing) to gain a consensus on an issue or problem. It is when physical meetings occur that people need to be most efficient and effective.

What does it do?

Effective meetings provide a forum to make necessary decisions and solve problems without wasting time. If meetings are effective, then something positive occurs, and there will be a result. People arrive on time, participate, offer information and ideas, and have a positive attitude. However, if meetings are not effective, people will often show up late, will be less likely to participate, and their attention and ideas will be less productive. To achieve effective meetings, treat them as processes, create standard rules to follow, and then adhere to those rules.

How do you do it?

The following steps or guidelines are used to run effective meetings:

1. Agree on a clear objective and agenda for the meeting.

2. Choose the right people for the meeting and notify everyone in advance.

---

3. Clarify roles and responsibilities for the meeting (i.e., leader, facilitator, scribe, timekeeper, technical representative, team member, etc.).

4. Ensure everyone adheres to meeting etiquette (being on time, turning off cell/smart phones, text messaging only during breaks, etc.).

5. Determine when face-to-face meetings are required, and, if and when additional meetings can be held via Web conferencing.

6. Evaluate the meetings regularly (at the end of the initial meeting and as needed) and improve the appropriate areas. *All meetings can be improved!*

7. Provide the list of Action Items to participants within 24 hours after the meeting.

The following are some common Web-based/Desktop sharing applications that can be used for meetings: Huddle.net, Zoho.com, WebEx.com, Google Drive (previously referred to as Google Docs), Groupsite.com, Zimbra.com, Gbidge.com, GoToMeeting.com, SharedView.com, etc.

The following benefits can be obtained by running effective meetings:

- ❖ Team members more likely to arrive on time and be engaged in the project
- ❖ Employees focused on the specific issue and "scope creep" is less likely to occur
- ❖ The likelihood of project completion may be sooner than expected
- ❖ Less time involved in the actual meetings
- ❖ Help to avoid stress on team members created by poorly managed meetings

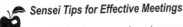

Sensei Tips for Effective Meetings

The following is an example on how one team evaluated their meetings:

Effective Meeting Evaluation Worksheet

Directions:
1. Spend only five minutes evaluating your meetings.
2. This form is most successful when everyone's responses are shared.
3. Focus on the weak spots, applaud the high ratings.

Rating System: Use the following 5-level Likert Item scale:
1 - Strongly Disagree
2 - Disagree
3 - Neither Agree nor Disagree
4 - Agree
5 - Strongly Agree

1	We stayed on the agenda.	3.6
2	We focused on the right issues during the meeting.	4.1
3	We focused on the issues and did not place blame.	4.3
4	Time was used wisely.	4.1
5	Information was presented accurately and clearly.	3.8
6	Everyone participated.	4.6
7	Action Items were assigned properly.	4.0
8	The pace of the meeting was appropriate.	3.6
9	Questions and concerns were addressed appropriately.	3.9
10	All ideas were explored given the time element.	4.2
	TOTAL:	40.2

Scoring Guidelines
45 - 50 Doing Well - Keep up the good work.
40 - 44 Doing OK - Must make more effort during meeting.
35 - 39 Not So Good - Must improve dramatically.

Once each team member completed their evaluation, the above team total of 40.2 was categorized as "Doing OK." Therefore, this group decided to improve evaluation item "(1) We stayed on the agenda." which was one of the lower scoring areas.

Effective Meetings

Project Management

Operations keep the lights on, strategy provides a light at the end of the tunnel, but project management is the train that moves the organization forward.
Joy Gumz

What is it?

Project management is the process of establishing, prioritizing, and carrying out tasks to complete specific objectives. This involves identifying and prioritizing tasks, identifying and assigning resources, in-process performance management of progress-to-outcomes, and taking actions to ensure success.

What does it do?

Program management is a broader topic and involves the process of managing multiple projects simultaneously in an on-going manner. Organizations may be simultaneously involved in program management of their Lean Sigma transformation and project management of several Lean Sigma improvement projects or initiatives.

Lean Sigma improvement projects are initiated from gaps identified in the assessment and gap analysis, gaps in performance metrics of actual performance to targeted requirements or expectations, improvement opportunities identified through value stream or process mapping activities, or market or regulatory driven projects to address customer needs and desires. It is critical to manage the resources needed to complete this work effectively. Organizations that initiate more projects than they can effectively support will find it difficult to succeed on a consistent basis. Resource management is a critical part of project management.

There are several popular project management tools. The most predominant tool for project and program management is the Gantt Chart, which is easily created in Excel. The other charts that are shown in this section can also easily be created in Excel with samples provided in the Sensei Tips for Project Management.

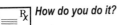

How do you do it?

The following steps or guidelines are used for good project management:

1. Describe the project in terms of overall objectives, measurements and activities, tasks, or events. Also define what is not included in the scope of the project. List the major pieces or steps of the project.

2. Assemble the project team and gain alignment on what was defined in (1) above.

3. Identify resources that will lead to successful project completion.

4. Construct a Gantt Chart showing the relationship/priorities between tasks and resources. List the minor or detailed steps (i.e., tasks) of the project. Include milestones to allow the team to get a sense of "mini-project" completion. This will reinforce the A3 or Lean Thinking that any and all improvements are possible.

5. Develop a time line and estimate due date targets and resources for each task (also referred to as the Action Item Log). *The Action Item (AI) Log is used by the team to assign and follow-up on specific actions items agreed to during the project.* The AI Log lists specific action items, the individual or group responsible to complete the action item, and when the action item is due to be completed. The AI Log can be used during regular team work sessions to follow-up on progress and to reassign resources and/or dates as necessary.

6. Shift resources and assign responsibilities as needed to meet the time line and quality objectives. Document ideas that may or may not be part of the current project by using an Issues and Opportunities Log. *The Issues and Opportunities (IO) Log is used by improvement teams to identify and document opportunities, ideas, issues, concerns, obstacles, roadblocks, and/or other items that the team is not quite sure what to do about.* The Issues and Opportunities Log is updated as items are identified and may have an indirect impact on Team Charter objectives. It is common for opportunities, ideas, and issues to arise during an improvement project. The IO Log acts as a holding place for opportunities and ideas that the team is not ready to act upon. Through periodic review and discussion, the team will observe that certain items from the IO Log are ready to be acted upon and subsequently move them from the IO Log to the AI Log and make the appropriate assignments.

7. Document and monitor progress on a regular basis relative to schedule, budget, and objectives. Make corrective actions as necessary.

The following benefits can be obtained by using good project management techniques:

- ❖ Improve efficiency and effectiveness completing the project
- ❖ Improve customer satisfaction (internal and/or external)
- ❖ Maximize employee's contributions and value-added work
- ❖ Identify opportunities to expand goods and services
- ❖ Allow for flexibility for project re-direction, if needed

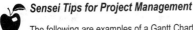

Sensei Tips for Project Management

The following are examples of a Gantt Chart, Action Items Log, and Issues and Opportunities Log:

Gantt Chart - Orthopedic Services Group

Objective: Record and track the key activities to complete the initiative. **Date:** June 28

Objective: Record and track action items

Team Name: Orthopedic Services Lean Sigma Improvement Team

Team Members: John, Linda, Sue, Greg, Brenda (core team)

■ Dark shading or green color signifies completed activities.
▢ Light shading or yellow color signifies on target.
△ Signifies behind schedule.
★ Denotes current week.

Prepare	Project Summary As Of 7/09	Week 1 2 3	★ 4	Week 5 6 7	8 9	Week 10 11 12
Lean Sigma Assessment	Completed					
Stakeholder Analysis	Completed					
Prioritize Projects	Completed					
Define Phase						
Create Team Charter	Completed					
Train everyone on teaming and project management	In progress					
Develop the current state map	In progress					
Collect process flow data	Behind schedule	△				
Measure Phase						
Collect Data	Not started					
Conduct Waste Walk	Not started					
Determine Demand Analysis	Not started					
Determine Process Capability	Not started					
Use MSA to create reliable measurement system	Not started					
Analyze Phase						
Develop Improvement Implementation Plan	Not started					
Complete a future state map	Not started					
Develop the detailed improvement plan for PDCAs	Not started					
Schedule 5 Days for PDCAs	Not started					

Action Item Log - Orthopedic Services Group

Objective: Record and track action items assigned to team members. **Revision Date:** July 22

Team Name: Orthopedic Services Lean Sigma Improvement Team

Team Members: John, Linda, Sue, Greg, Brenda (core team members)

	Action Item - Task Description	Who	Start Date	Expected Completion	Completion Date	Comments
1	John to meet with Linda to review Team Charter and meeting times.	John	28 Jun	29 Jun	29 Jun	
2	Conduct assessment and provide information to team.	Linda	1 Jul	6 Jul	8 Jul	Staff unavailable.
3	Finalize Team Charter (ensure new patient exam times are included).	Sue	30 Jun	1 Jul	1 Jul	
4	Sub-team of Greg, Linda, and Sue to complete initial current state map.	Greg	4 Jul	8 Jul	8 Jul	
5	Team review current state map.	Team	18 Jul	18 Jul	18 Jul	
6	Gather additional data for current state map.	Brenda	7 Jul	14 Jul	10 Jul	
7	Obtain demand analysis data for last 6 months (new patients only).	Sue	7 Jul	8 Jul	10 Jul	Data incomplete.
8	Obtain new patient scheduling data.	Brenda	10 Jul	12 Jul	11 Jul	
9	Organize all data in appropriate charts for review.	Greg	10 Jul	12 Jul	11 Jul	
10	Communicate to staff first part of team's progress.	Linda	14 Jul	14 Jul	14 Jul	
11	Obtain overtime numbers from Jenny.	Linda	10 Jul	10 Jul	10 Jul	
12	Obtain patient complaint history for last 6 months (new patients only).	Greg	28 Jun	7 Jul	9 Jul	
13	Complete current state map.	Team	8 Jul	10 Jul	14 Jul	Too busy.
14	Begin Analyze Phase.	Team	22 Jul	14 Aug		

Issues and Opportunities Log - Orthopedic Services Group

Objective: Record and track Opportunities (O), Ideas (I), Roadblocks (RB), and Parking Lot (PL) items.   **Revision Date:** June 28

Team Name: Orthopedic Services Lean Sigma Improvement Team

Team Members: John, Linda, Sue, Greg, Brenda (core team members)

Medium shading or green color signifies moved to Action Item Log.

What is In Question?	Category (O/I/RB/PL)	Assigned To	Date Logged	Date Addressed	Comments
Should someone from IT attend all sessions?	I	John	28 Jun	1 Jul	Larry from IT to attend monthly meetings, with weekly updates.
We need immediate data on all aspects of new patients.	I	Linda	28 Jun		Save for new team.
Need to improve scheduling for all patients, not just new exams.	O	Greg	14 Jul		Save for new team.
We need more parking space in the rear of the building.	PL	John	14 Jul		Out-of-scope.
We are too busy to meet every week!	RB	Sue	14 Jul	14 Jul	Continue to meet.
Team Charter to include goal to reduce new patient exam times.	O	Linda	28 Jun	1 Jul	Move to AI Log. (Item #3)
The patient complaint field is not functioning, need IT involvement.	RB	Greg	22 Jul		Submit IT request.
We need to standardize new exams and monitor progress.	I	Sue	22 Jul		On hold for later.
Hire part-time PA to work weekends to extend service hours.	I	Judy	22 Jul		On hold for later.

The statement "Team Charter to include goal to reduce new patient exam times." was added to (3) Action Item Log (previous page).

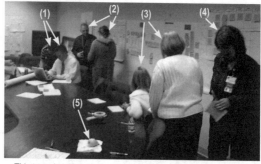

This team is in Day 2 of a Standard 5 Day Kaizen Event. Good project management techniques are demonstrated. Everyone has specific assignments. Note the following: (1) team members analyzing data and creating appropriate charts, (2) team members discussing where to take photos (typically done in Day 1), (3) team members reviewing the value stream map, (4) team member going to the process area, and (5) team member having left their healthy snack! This team is very productive and is making great progress.

Value Stream and Process Maps
(w/ SIPOC Diagram)

If you find a path with no obstacles, it
probably doesn't lead anywhere.
Fred A. Clark

What is it?

A **value stream map** is a visual representation of the material, work, and information flow, as well as the queue times between processes for a specific customer demand. The value stream map is a very powerful tool and does an excellent job highlighting wastes (i.e., delays, excess transport, etc.) for processes.

What does it do?

A current state value stream map provides a representation of how the process is currently running. A future state value stream map represents the process with the proposed improvements that are to be implemented. The future state value stream map is a road map for improvement. It is recommended that a current state value stream map be drawn on a whiteboard or on a long sheet of white paper that can be hung on the wall. Post-it Notes can then represent various activities within a process. If a long sheet of paper is not available, tape multiple flip chart sheets on the wall and line them up horizontally. Number each flip chart sheet to ensure they stay organized once the event is over.

Most current state value stream mapping exercises are done on paper that is posted on the wall. This means there may be waste involved if the team desires to subsequently recreate the map electronically using Visio or Excel, or some other flow charting application. However, that type of waste is minimal compared to the benefits of employee engagement and what that can provide. Do not underestimate the importance of employee engagement!

The following steps or guidelines are used to create a value stream map:

1. Use the following icons to draw a "shell" of the current state, listing the main processes, customers, and suppliers (internal and external). Consider creating additional icons that may be appropriate to your value stream (e.g., creating a laptop icon to demonstrate interactivity with the Customer Relationship Management (CRM) system).

Dedicated Process Box - the main process, department, or area where value-added and/or non value-added work occurs

Shared Process Box - where multiple value streams all inter-relate (mail rooms, human resources, billing, lab admissions, lobby areas, pharmacy, etc.)

Attribute Area - characteristics of the process (e.g., cycle times, number of employees, internal defects, etc.)

Customer or Supplier - the upstream and downstream customer or supplier, with its respective attributes or characteristics

External Transport - the physical arrival or departure of the patient related to the value stream (car, EMT, MED-flight, etc.)

Queue (Wait) Time - the amount of time, work, patients, supplies, or information that resides between two processes

Database/Internet Interaction - computer interaction (e.g., EMR, email, Web, etc.)

Manual Information Flow - physical conveyance of work, employees, or customers between two processes (e.g., hand carrying work to another area, transporting patients, etc.)

Electronic Information Flow - the electronic signal that communicates information

Mail - the arrival or sending of metered mail

Email - the arrival or sending of email

Folder - a single unit of work (i.e., document, chart, labs, etc.)

Folders - multiple work units grouped together and moved through a common process

Go-See Scheduling - the physical viewing and collecting of information on processes to determine workloads (e.g., patients backed up, etc.)

Push - the movement of the patient, performance of service or work, or information transmission *regardless of need* of the downstream process or activity

Staff - the person assigned to the particular process

Measurement - the process metric

Hassle Factor - (not to be confused with David Hasselhoff ☺) - indicates high hassle factor/frustration level for the customer

Smiley Face - indicates customer/patient satisfaction or delight options

Note: If there is any confusion about processes used to create the value stream map, consider creating a SIPOC Diagram. *A **SIPOC Diagram** is a tool used by a team to identify all relevant elements of a process improvement project or identified value stream to help ensure all aspects of the process are taken into consideration and that no key components are missing.* SIPOC is an acronym for the Suppliers (the 'S' in SIPOC) of the process, the Inputs (I) to the process, the Process (P) that is under review, the Outputs (O) of the process, and the Customers (C) that receive the process outputs. The following is an example of a SIPOC Diagram:

SIPOC Chart
Laboratory
Specimen Flow

Process

Inputs
Patient
Medical History
Tx Facilities
Patient Condition
Registration Info
Insurance Verify
Physician Licensed
Physician
Requisition

Process Flow →
Order Entry
Collection
Delivery
Processing
Testing
Report
Notification

Outputs
Electronic/Hard Copy
Bill
Accurate Result
Stored Specimen
Critical Result Phone
Stored Orders
Calibration Reports
Completed Worksheets

Suppliers
Physician Office
ER
Physicians in house
Insurance Companies
Off-site Hospitals
Patient
Couriers

Customers
Patients
Nurses
Doctors/Offices
Payors
Lab

Trigger
Physician Writes Order

Done
Physician Reads Result

Define

Value Stream and Process Maps (w/ SIPOC Diagram)

2. Visit the areas, beginning with the most downstream process and walk the flow in reverse order to collect the attributes (i.e., cycle times, defects, etc.) related to the value stream and, if applicable, gather actual data. Use a stopwatch (if practical) and clearly communicate to everyone in the area what you are doing and why. This may also be the time to conduct the Waste Walk while you are visiting the area. (See Waste Walk in the Measure Phase.)

3. Determine the amount of time between processes. This is the main determinant on the separation of process boxes on a value stream map. If delays are occurring within processes more than a certain percentage (e.g., 10% of the overall lead time), then that may warrant a separation of those processes on a value stream map. (Later, additional tools will be used to further analyze these delays within the process.)

4. Determine the quantity of work that arrives at each process (i.e., # of reports, labs, patients, interruptions per hour, etc.).

5. Determine what is done with the work after the process has been completed. What is the next process? Does anything special need to be done prior to the work arriving at the next process?

6. List all the process attributes on the current state map. If there are other departmental or process attributes (i.e., cycle time of the activities, # of patients seen, errors/defects/mistakes, etc.) specific to the process, list those as appropriate.

7. Draw all forms of communication, electronic and/or manual.

8. Sum the process cycle times within the process box. This is typically the value-added time which may include some of the non value-added time due to a poor process (which can be later analyzed for waste). If delays are listed within the process attributes, then it would be acceptable to include those delays within the total process cycle time. Additional Lean Sigma tools will be used to separate and eliminate those wastes; however, many times the larger waste of time (i.e., delay) will be between the processes. There is no right or wrong method to list delays, just be consistent in your approach when mapping.

9. Compile a step graph at the bottom of the value stream map displaying the total cycle time for each process, including the queue/wait/delay times.

10. Brainstorm with the team and create a first pass future state using the following icons:

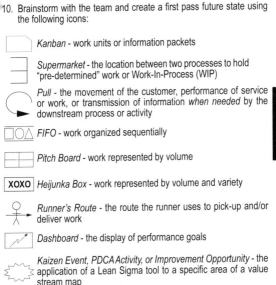

Kanban - work units or information packets

Supermarket - the location between two processes to hold "pre-determined" work or Work-In-Process (WIP)

Pull - the movement of the customer, performance of service or work, or transmission of information *when needed* by the downstream process or activity

FIFO - work organized sequentially

Pitch Board - work represented by volume

Heijunka Box - work represented by volume and variety

Runner's Route - the route the runner uses to pick-up and/or deliver work

Dashboard - the display of performance goals

Kaizen Event, PDCA Activity, or Improvement Opportunity - the application of a Lean Sigma tool to a specific area of a value stream map

This is a sample of common icons used in value stream mapping; organizations should create additional industry specific icons as appropriate.

Note: Visio and Excel are common applications to create value stream and process maps. There are others such as SmartDraw, Smooth Flowcharter, FlowBreeze, ConceptDraw, SigmaFlow, iBrainstorming, etc. Many of these allow a 30-day trial prior to purchasing.

Note: The following value stream and process maps under Sensei Tips are reduced images and the text details are not the focus. Each map is noted at the bottom for its uniqueness. The larger image of these can be obtained by requesting the page number to info@ theleanstore.com.

Sensei Tips for Value Stream Mapping

The following are examples of value stream maps and value stream mapping sessions:

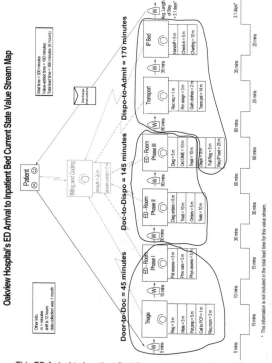

This ED Arrival to Inpatient Bed Current State Value Stream Map has identified three sub-value streams within the overall stream. This allowed the team to coordinate improvements and manage the improvement project better by having three separate mini Kaizen Events.

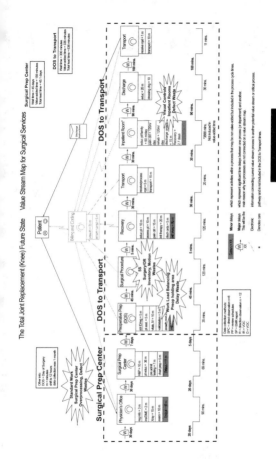

*This Total Joint Replacement (Knee) Future State Value Stream Map
includes numerous Kaizen Events to meet the team's objectives.*

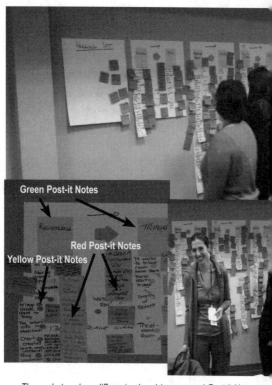

These photos show different colored (see arrows) Post-it Notes being used to identify the various processes and activities for a value stream. Green represents main processes such as Triage, front desk, registration, etc.), yellow represents tasks within work areas, red represents wastes or bottlenecks in the process. Mapping can be fun! (Also, these employees may have invested in Post-it Notes.)

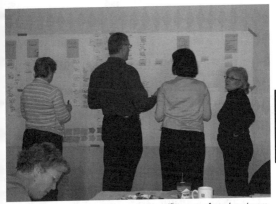

These team members are discussing specific areas of a value stream map. Once the current state has been documented, then Lean Six Sigma tools can be used to create a future state (map) free of process waste and variation.

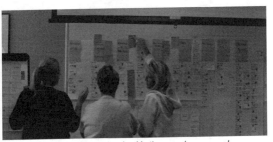

Get employees involved in the mapping process!

What is it?

A **process map (or flowchart)** is a visual representation of a series of operations (tasks, activities) consisting of people, work duties, and transactions that occur in the delivery of a product or service. Note: In this book, process maps and flowcharts are used interchangeably.

The project team should tackle the mapping activity as if it were doing an investigation (find out exactly what is and is not happening in the process). Process maps use standard symbols to represent an operation, process, and/or set of tasks to be performed which provides a common language for the project team to visualize problems. It also allows for the process to be easier to read and understand, thus making it a visual tool to see areas of waste, process variation, and/or redundancy.

What does it do?

The following are the main five types of flowcharts that will assist you to visualize the process:

1. **Basic process maps (macro level)** identify all the major steps in a process - usually no more than six steps. They are mostly used for the "30,000 foot view" for management review.

2. **Basic process maps (micro level)** examine the process in detail and indicate all the steps or activities (i.e., the decision points, waiting periods, tasks that must be redone (rework), and any feedback loops). This is the "ground level" listing of process activities.

3. **Deployment process maps** (also referred to as Swim Lane maps) examine the process in terms of who is carrying out the steps, and is conveyed in the form of a matrix, showing the various participants and the flow of steps among these participants. These maps are helpful if the process crosses departmental boundaries.

4. **Opportunity process maps** examine the activities that create the process and list differences between value-added and non value-added activities.

5. **Spaghetti diagram process maps** use a continuous line to trace the path of an item, document, person, or service that is being provided through all its phases. Spaghetti diagrams expose inefficient layouts and large distances traveled between steps. These diagrams should also display electronic information flow (emails, spreadsheets, documents, etc.).

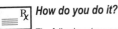

How do you do it?

The following steps or guidelines are used to create a process map:

1. Identify the right people needed to develop the process map. This may require people from outside the project team for their expertise and knowledge. These are Subject Matter Experts (SMEs).

2. Define the process boundaries with the beginning and ending points of the process. Define required process inputs.

3. Define the level of detail and type of map required.

4. Use the following standard icons to represent the processes and activities for a current state process map.

Ovals represent the beginning and ending points of a process.

Rectangles are used to describe an action or a task.

Diamonds contain questions that require a "Yes" or "No" decision and indicate appropriate process flow.

Partial pages represent a document.

Multiple partial pages represent a report or an output with multiple documents.

→ Arrows represent the direction of process flow.

Queue symbols represent a delay in the process.

Rectangles with drop shadows represent that a more detailed flowchart of the process exists.

Modified rectangles represent a standard, protocol, or SOP.

Triangles represent a process measurement.

Rounded rectangles represent a meeting, conference call, or Webinar.

Circles represent where the flow continues onto a different page or to another process.

Value Stream and Process Maps (w/ SIPOC Diagram) 67

5. Brainstorm with the team and create a first pass future state using Lean Sigma tools and concepts.

6. Circulate the map to other people within the process for input and/or clarification and update as needed.

The following benefits can be obtained by creating a value stream or process map:

❖ Allow all stakeholders to "see" the entire process at-a-glance
❖ Serve as a visual inventory for improvements
❖ Help to achieve consensus for improvement ideas

Whatever type of process map is created, use the following sequence of steps to further analyze the process being examined:

1. Examine each process for bottlenecks, redundancy or unnecessary steps, lack of capacity, weak links, poorly-defined steps, cost added-only steps, rework, poor quality (error prone activity), etc.

2. Examine each activity, loop back, or decision symbol to determine if it can be streamlined or removed.

A hospital can be enormously complex. Only visuals can convey enough information to understand the complex process dependencies and hidden waste. A visualization tool, such as the value stream or process map, provides a deeper understanding of these complex processes allowing for major breakthroughs in improving the patient experience. It is a prolific change management tool that leads to a consensus on systemic problems and remedies. Visualization through mapping allows greater insight into process improvement, shifts in paradigms, and it builds consensus through staff engagement – changing the way business is conducted.

Value stream and process maps take different perspectives, but, they both help visualize areas for improvement. While no mapping technique fits every situation and purpose, the following can be used as a guide:

Use a value stream map when:
- ❖ You need to show major process steps to provide a broader and wider view
- ❖ Processes are fairly sequential with no more than 3 - 5 decision trees identified
- ❖ No more than 10 processes/work cells need to be mapped
- ❖ Material and information flow needs to be visually displayed – this is true for both
- ❖ Waste needs to be identified from the customer's perspective (value-added versus non value-added activities)
- ❖ Flow is an issue
- ❖ Key metrics need to be reviewed (i.e., cycle times, defect rates, wait/delay times, productivity, inventory levels, changeover times, etc.)
- ❖ Delays between processes need highlighting
- ❖ The focus has to be from the customer's perspective

Use a process map when:
- ❖ Processes may or may not be sequential
- ❖ Tasks are done in parallel
- ❖ Multiple decision points need to be identified
- ❖ No limit to processes being mapped
- ❖ A thorough understanding of the process is required
- ❖ Developing a training program
- ❖ Extraneous activities or tasks need to be highlighted
- ❖ The focus needs to be on the tasks or activities

Define

Sensei Tips for Process Mapping

The following are examples of process maps:

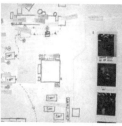

This Spaghetti Diagram included photos to help understand the process. Photos will assist team members to better connect to the processes. They may also "trigger" additional input as to wasteful activities as well as ways to eliminate those wastes.

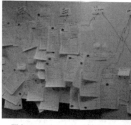

This mapping exercise consisted of posting screen shots of their EMR system helping them see many "overprocessing" wastes (repeat data entry, extra data, etc.). Just because the process is automated it does not mean it is without waste!

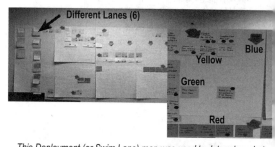

This Deployment (or Swim Lane) map was used to determine what needed to be integrated into the new EMR system. The large arrows (Blue) identified wastes, make electronic (Green), keep as is (Yellow), and needs protocol (Red). The dots represented various process improvements in progress.

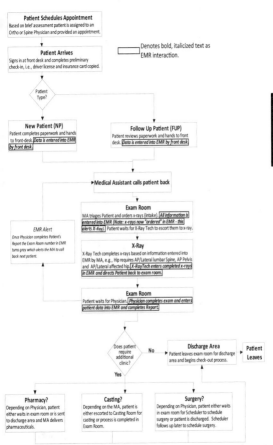

Patient Schedules Appointment
Based on brief assessment patient is assigned to an Ortho or Spine Physician and provided an appointment.

Patient Arrives
Signs in at front desk and completes preliminary check-in, i.e., driver license and insurance card copied.

Denotes bold, italicized text as EMR interaction.

Patient Type?

New Patient (NP)
Patient completes paperwork and hands to front-desk. *Data is entered into EMR by front desk.*

Follow Up Patient (FUP)
Patient reviews paperwork and hands to front desk. *Data is entered into EMR by front desk.*

►Medical Assistant calls patient back

EMR Alert
Once Physician completes Patient's Report the Exam Room number in EMR turns grey which alerts the MA to call back next patient.

Exam Room
MA triages Patient and orders x-rays (intake). *All information is entered into EMR (Note: x-rays now "ordered" in EMR - this alerts X-Ray).* Patient waits for X-Ray Tech to escort them to x-ray.

X-Ray
X-Ray Tech completes x-rays based on information entered into EMR by MA, e.g., Hip requires AP/Lateral lumbar Spine, AP Pelvis and AP/Lateral affected hip. *X-RayTech enters completed x-rays in EMR and directs Patient back to exam room.*

Exam Room
Patient waits for Physician. *Physician completes exam and enters patient data into EMR and completes Report.*

Does patient require additional clinic?

No → **Discharge Area**
Patient leaves exam room for discharge area and begins check-out process. → **Patient Leaves**

Yes

Pharmacy?
Depending on Physician, patient either waits in exam room or is sent to discharge area and MA delivers pharmaceuticals.

Casting?
Depending on the MA, patient is either escorted to Casting Room for casting or process is completed in Exam Room.

Surgery?
Depending on Physician, patient either waits in exam room for Scheduler to schedule surgery or patient is discharged. Scheduler follows up later to schedule surgery.

This basic process map (micro level) is the Patient Experience Current State Process Map. The bold, italicized text denotes EMR interaction. Teams need to be creative to map complex processes.

Define

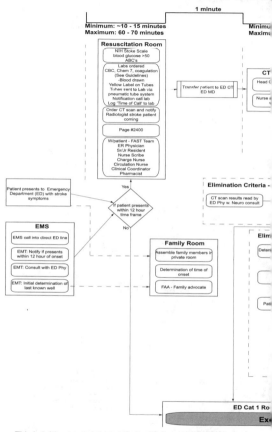

GOAL: Total Tin

1 minute

Minimum: ~10 - 15 minutes
Maximum: 60 - 70 minutes

Minimu
Maximu

Resuscitation Room

NIH Stroke Scale
blood glucose >50
ABC's

Labs ordered
CBC, Chem 7, coagulation
(See Guidelines)
-Blood drawn
Yellow Label on Tubes
Tubes sent to Lab via
pneumatic tube system
Notification call lab
Log 'Time of Call' to lab

Order CT scan and notify
Radiologist stroke patient
coming

Page #2400

W/patient - FAST Team
ER Physician
Sr/Jr Resident
Nurse Scribe
Charge Nurse
Circulation Nurse
Clinical Coordinator
Pharmacist

Transfer patient to ED OT
ED MD

CT

Head C

Nurse

Patient presents to Emergency
Department (ED) with stroke
symptoms

If patient presents
within 12 hour
time frame

Yes

No

Elimination Criteria -

CT scan results read by
ED Phy w. Neuro consult

Elim

Deter

EMS

EMS call into direct ED line

EMT: Notify if presents
within 12 hour of onset

EMT: Consult with ED Phy

EMT: Initial determination of
last known well

Family Room

Assemble family members in
private room

Determination of time of
onset

FAA - Family advocate

Deter

Pati

ED Cat 1 Ro

Ex

*This hybrid current state map is for the Door-to-Needle for Primary
Stroke Certification value stream. Colors (not shown) were used to
denote the various sections.*

from ED Door to Needle < 60 minutes

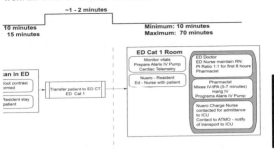

~1 - 2 minutes

10 minutes
15 minutes

Minimum: 10 minutes
Maximum: 70 minutes

:an in ED

/out contrast
ormed

Resident stay
patient

Transfer patient to ED CT
ED Cat 1

ED Cat 1 Room

Monitor vitals
Prepare Alaris IV Pump
Cardiac Telemetry

Nuero - Resident
Ed - Nurse with patient

ED Doctor
ED Nurse maintain RN:
Pt Ratio 1:1 for first 8 hours
Pharmacist

Pharmacist
Mixes IV-tPA (5-7 minutes)
Hang IV
Programs Alaris IV Pump

Nuero Charge Nurse
contacted for admittance
to ICU
Contact to ATMO - notify
of transport to ICU

Define

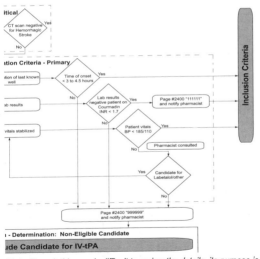

itical

CT scan negative
for Hemorrhagic
Stroke — Yes

No

tion Criteria - Primary

tion of last known
well — Time of onset
< 3 to 4.5 hours — Yes

No

ab results — Lab results
negative patient on
Coumadin
INR < 1.7 — Yes — Page #2400 "111111"
and notify pharmacist

No

vitals stabilized — Patient vitals
BP < 185/110 — Yes

No — Pharmacist consulted

Yes — Candidate for
Labetalol/other

No

Page #2400 "999999"
and notify pharmacist

Inclusion Criteria

- Determination: Non-Eligible Candidate

ude Candidate for IV-tPA

Note: Though this map is difficult to review the details, its purpose is to demonstrate the uniqueness of the main process areas and how the data was recorded.

Value Stream and Process Maps (w/ SIPOC Diagram)   73

Lean Thinking Statements for the Define Phase

The following Lean Thinking Statement assessment should be done as an individual and, if desired, combined and discussed as a team. If the team leader realizes that many of the items are an issue for certain team members, then maybe a one-on-one with those specific individuals would be appropriate. Or, if a few of the team members have similar concerns over one or two of the statements, then possibly these should be addressed with the team. Continue with open and honest dialogue with the team. As a team member, it is YOUR responsibility to address any of the statements that hinder YOUR individual input to the team's progress. These statements are not to be taken lightly!

Use the 5 Level Likert Scale for the following statements:

> 1 - Strongly Disagree
> 2 - Disagree
> 3 - Neither Agree nor Disagree
> 4 - Agree
> 5 - Strongly Agree

I am in agreement with the Team Charter. _____
I believe we have the right people on the team. _____
The meetings have been productive. _____
The value stream (or process) map helped to identify wastes. _____
I participated in the meetings. _____
Action items have been assigned equitably. _____
I am confident in discussing this project with my colleagues. _____
I see the value in this team's approach. _____
I believe I can add value to this team. _____
I believe my ideas will be heard and considered. _____

Total Score: _____

If your score is less than 80% (40 points), then more work should be completed before moving on to the Measure Phase. Ensure A3 Project Report Sections 1. Problem Statement and 2. Current State are nearly completed.

Note: The Value Stream and Process Map will likely be used again in the A3 Project Report Section 5. Future State.

The Measure Phase

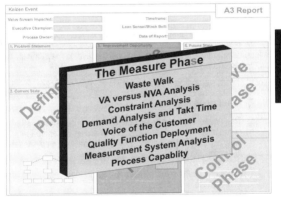

The Measure Phase

Waste Walk
VA versus NVA Analysis
Constraint Analysis
Demand Analysis and Takt Time
Voice of the Customer
Quality Function Deployment
Measurement System Analysis
Process Capablity

Tools listed in this section are most likely to be used at this time. All the tools can be applicable at any phase of a Kaizen Project as determined by the needs of the project team.

Waste Walk

Be a yardstick of quality. Some people aren't used to an environment where excellence is expected.
Steve Jobs

What is it?

A **Waste Walk** is an activity when project team members visit a process area that is being considered for improvement, ask questions, and then identify the wastes on the current state value stream or process map. Many of the team members will be very familiar with the project area as it is their actual work area. Conducting this Waste Walk, the team members, along with their Lean Sigma training, will be viewing their areas with a fresh perspective as they look at the processes and work flows.

Note: The Waste Walk can also be done in the Analyze Phase.

What does it do?

The Waste Walk is typically done after an initial value stream or process map has been created. It allows the entire team to "see" the process real-time. The Waste Walk accomplishes the following:

❖ Ensure everyone is aligned to the physical location of the processes analyzed
❖ Ensure process workers are engaged in improvement activities
❖ Allow for all process workers to provide input
❖ Allow for open communications about the team's project
❖ Allow for discussions about the process to clear up any questions

How do you do it?

The following steps or guidelines are used to conduct a Waste Walk:

1. Educate the team members on the following wastes as well as suggested questions to detect waste.

Overproduction - Producing some type of work prior to it being required is waste of overproduction. Providing a quality product or service above and beyond what is needed is also considered overproduction. Overproduction is when too much of something is made or served. This is the greatest of all the wastes. Overproduction of work or services can cause other wastes.

To DETECT this waste ask:

Is service required faster or slower than takt time (or demand)?
Is there inventory (i.e., supplies, patients, orders, labs, reports, etc.) in a queue waiting to be processed immediately downstream?
Is there a lack of continuous flow?
Is work scheduled according to a schedule?
Is a pull system being used?
Is takt time or demand known?

Waiting - Waiting for anything (people, signatures, information, etc.) is waste. This waste of waiting is "low hanging fruit" which is easy to reach and ripe for the taking. Waiting means idle time and that causes workflow to stop. We often do not think of paper sitting in an In-basket or an unread email as waste. However, when looking for the item (document or email), how many times do we mull through that In-basket or the Inbox folder to try to find it? How many times do you actually touch something before it is completed? The finish it, file it, or throw it away system helps eliminate this waste.

To DETECT this waste ask:

Am I just watching the same process and not adding value or contributing to any improvements?
Can something else be completed that is value-added while I am waiting?
Is standardized work being following?
Are there "buffers" between processes for a reason? And, if so, have there been any ideas on how the "buffers" can be reduced or eliminated?
Are Kanbans being used effectively?
Does the transport time seem excessive?
Are performance or operational measures being met?
Are performance or operational measures being improved upon?

Motion - Any movement or unnecessary motion of people, material, supplies, documents, etc. that does not add value is waste. This waste is created by poor physical layout or design, faulty or outdated equipment, supply inaccessibility, and movement of information or data that does not add value. The waste of motion is insidious and is hidden in old procedures that have not been reviewed for continuous improvement initiatives. Regardless of the industry, motion waste may appear as someone who is looking "busy" but not adding value to the work or service.

To DETECT this waste ask:

> Can walking or excess movement of work, patient, or employee be reduced?
> Can body movement be reduced?
> Are shortcuts being used to reduce keystrokes for data and information input and/or retrieval?
> Is the work area optimized for ease of work and ergonomic reasons?
> Is there an active 5S program?
> Is standard work being followed and improved upon?
> Is cross-training being done?

Transport - Transport waste is the excess movement of people, materials, supplies, documents, information, etc. within an organization. Excess transport affects the delivery of any work or service within an organization. Even with the Internet and email readily available, too often, or not often enough, documents (i.e., files) or products that provide little or no value are moved downstream regardless of need. Reducing or eliminating excess transport waste is important. Locating all work in sequential process operations and as physically close together as possible will help eliminate or reduce this waste. Transport between processes that cannot be eliminated should be automated as much as possible. Ask questions such as: *Is the physical layout optimal?, Is the release and request for work automated?, and Is IT aware of the problem and can they help?"*

To DETECT this waste ask:

> Are supplies or work being stored in inventory of some sort?
> Is the physical layout causing unnecessary transportation needs?
> Is the communication of work transfer automated and does it only move if the downstream process signals for it?
> Are there any obstacles to transportation such as detours, inventory in the way, transport unavailability (breakdown, inaccessibility, lost, etc.)?

Overprocessing - Putting more effort into the work than what is required by internal or external customers is waste. This waste is going above and beyond the needs and expectations of the customer. Many people see this waste as improved quality, but it is not. Quality is meeting needs and expectations. Excessive processing does not add value.

To DETECT this waste ask:

Is this a poor process design and what is its purpose?
Are incorrect process capabilities specified?
Is the process or service building excessive quality into the product or service to compensate for downstream process or service failure?
Is there a clear understanding of the customer/patient requirements?
Is someone doing the same process but differently?
Is standard work defined?

Inventory - Excessive piles of supplies, paperwork, computer files (e.g., emails) are the waste of inventory and cause extra time searching. They all take up space or require someone's time to stock and search if not organized. If work is accumulating or backing up between processes, waste of inventory is present. Work-In-Process (WIP) may be an asset, but it is waste.

To DETECT this waste ask:

Are there queues throughout the value stream or processes?
Is there obsolete inventory?
Is the process capable?
Is standard work being followed and improved upon?
Is there too much variation in the process?

Defect - Defect waste refers to all processing required in creating a defect and the additional work required to correct a defect or error. Defects and errors (either internal or external) result in additional processing that add no value to the product or service. It takes less time to do work correctly the first time than the time it would take to do it over. Rework or correction of work is waste and adds more cost to any product or service for which the customer will not pay. This waste can reduce profits significantly.

To DETECT this waste ask:

What is the capability (variation from specification) or sigma value (defect rate) for the process?
Are there common reasons for the defects?

People's Skills - The underutilization of people is a result of not placing people where they can (and will) use their knowledge, skills, and abilities to their fullest potential providing value-added work and services. An effective performance management system will reduce this waste significantly.

To DETECT this waste ask:

Are employees effectively cross-trained?
Are employees encouraged to suggest improvements?
Are new employees trained to best practice before they begin working?
Are employees improving the work standard?

Unevenness - Lack of a consistent flow of inputs/information/scheduled work from upstream processes causes many other types of waste. Waste of unevenness creates fluctuations in workloads and unbalanced services and impacts other processes. This waste directly impacts customers and can cause frustration for employees.

To DETECT this waste ask:

Are employees effectively cross-trained?
Is work scheduled to the day or hour?
Are employees aware of the next process requirements?
Are there times when work piles up in front of a particular process?
Have bottlenecks and/or constraints been identified?

Overburden - Overburdening or overloading occurs when the capacity of the process is not known and/or is not adequately scheduled. This typically causes other wastes to occur. Overburden must be handled as a separate waste; it can be identified easily during the value mapping process and is often expressed in terms of capacities of equipment or people. Usually this waste causes a great sense of frustration, anger, and job dissatisfaction on the part of the employee. This most likely would have a negative impact on the customer as well.

To DETECT this waste ask:

Are employees effectively cross-trained?
Is capacity known for all processes?
Does customer demand vary and is capacity flexible to the changes?
Is work scheduled through multiple processes with standard times?
Is standard work being followed for repetitive tasks?

Environmental Resources - As organizations become more sustainable or "Green," they have to make extra efforts to protect environmental resources. Any waste generated by an organization that negatively impacts the environment, whether it is solid or liquid, is classified as environmental waste.

To DETECT this waste ask:

Are employees aware of environmental waste?
Are there supplies or materials that have a reusable alternative or recycled potential?
Are there any forms of recycling being done now?

Social Responsibility - Social Responsibility waste is broad and includes poverty, discrimination, health and injuries, nutrition, literacy and education, office politics, and social media networking.

To DETECT this waste ask:

Are employees aware of personal communication rules during work time?
Are social networks (Facebook, Twitter, etc.) being used to promote the services to the appropriate market segment?
Are employees ethical in how business is being conducted?
Is training conducted regularly on diversification in the workplace?

(Waste Walk - How to Do It? Continued)

2. Communicate to the employees working in the prospective areas/ processes/departments when you will be bringing the group through and explain your purpose using an "elevator speech." *An elevator speech is a brief, comprehensive verbal overview on the purpose and related activities regarding the product, process, or service being examined.* It should convey the following: *"Here's what our project is about............," "Here's why it's important to do............," "Here's what success will look like............," and "Here's what we need from you.......... ."*

3. Assign one person in each group to take notes. Use the Waste Walk Checlist example on the following page as a guide. This can easily be created in Microsoft Excel or Word. It is also available at www. TheLeanStore.com for a nominal fee.

4. Ensure the team has thought of questions to ask, including: What are some of the issues affecting your work? What could be improved? Do you help out when things get busy? If not, why? Do you know when you are behind schedule? Do you know when the work you provide is needed downstream (or the next process)? It is suggested you review the "To DETECT this waste ask:" parts for each waste and create a set of 3 – 6 questions.

5. Do not cause any disruption to the process. (e.g., If a Waste Walk is to be conducted through the Emergency Department of a hospital, if possible, schedule a walk during the least busy or slack time.)

6. If the group is larger than 5, break into smaller groups.

7. Start with the last downstream process and work backwards upstream.

8. Thank the people for their time.

9. Consolidate the information from the Waste Walk and update the current state value stream or process map with how these wastes can be reduced or eliminated through the use of Lean Sigma tools and concepts. This will be further referenced in the Improve Phase.

The following benefits can be obtained by conducting a Waste Walk:

❖ Provide additional insight into processes that are being examined
❖ Connect classroom value stream or process mapping to the actual processes
❖ Allow for everyone to "see" or walk the process flow to all be on the same page

Note: If program applications are being analyzed for electronic waste, consider either having the appropriate screen shots or the application available for the team to review.

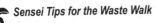

Sensei Tips for the Waste Walk

The following is an example of an elevator speech as well as information derived from a Waste Walk:

"Our project, ED Throughput, is a group effort to improve the efficiency of our process while decreasing the length of patient stay in the ED. It's important to increase our customers' satisfaction and confidence in our services. When we're successful, we improve associate satisfaction while reaching our target of 2.5 hours in the ED (or less). We need you to have an open mind and to accept any future changes that we may make." (Treat to Street!)

ER Waste Walk Sheet				
Waste Category	Observation	Possible Solutions from People Doing the Work	Impact on Value Stream Performance	Value Stream "problem"
Defects: Equipment failure of missing, incomplete information		Better equipment, TP in triage	Small impact	Doing the work
Overproduction: I could not find any evidence of overproduction.				
Waiting: Waiting for patient to get registered. pt's recalling meds, needed to redirect patient to stay on task during triage. Registration not quick reg all patients.		Pulling info forward. Given patients wallet insert to keep meds on. Quick reg out front, finish reg in the back.	Big impact	Making work flow
Not Utilizing Employees: Security underutilized with regards to control of lobby and visitors. Volunteers to help patients into ER and up to front desk.		Security to control lobby with a volunteer assisting patients and visitors.	Big impact	Doing the work
Transportation: Moving patients back to beds that are dirty, thus moving them again.		Flagging dirty beds.	Moderate impact	Making work flow
Inventory: Patients waiting to see triage nurse, and ultimately the doctor.		Charge nurse perform as a relief valve.	Moderate impact	Making work flow
Motion: Searching for equipment (one touch, temporal thermometer) Poor layout requiring nurse to open door and push wheelchair at same time.		Redesign triage area with more equipment.	Small impact	Making work flow
Extra Processing: Doctors and nurses asking the patient the same questions. Overlap with DR and RN exam. EKG LOG		Teamwork approach.	Small impact	Doing the work

This ED improvement team asked two docs (one shown in this example), the ED Director, and the ED Manager to complete the ER Waste Walk Sheet after the team conducted their Waste Walk. Their issues (i.e., wastes) were addressed as the team moved forward.

Measure

Value-Added (VA) versus Non Value-Added (NVA) Analysis

It's not so much how busy you are, but why you are busy. The bee is praised. The mosquito is swatted.
Marie O'Connor

What is it?

The **VA versus NVA Analysis** is used to illuminate the waste in a process. Once the process steps are documented by a value stream or process map, VA and NVA times can be measured and placed into a simple data table to compare the Value-Added (VA) to Non Value-Added (NVA) time content for a portion (one process) of the value stream or for all the processes at the system level.

What does it do?

The VA versus NVA Analysis is a form of a time study. When conducting time studies, do not be overly concerned with whether the time is from the fastest or slowest person. Take accurate measurements and document them. If there is concern regarding the relative speed (or lack thereof) for an individual process, simply document the concern. The fact that there is this concern over the possible variation in times will lead to discussions and will very well lead to key process improvements.

How do you do it?

The following steps or guidelines are used to conduct a VA versus NVA Analysis:

1. List process steps to be analyzed in a spreadsheet program.

2. Create a table with the following category labels. (See example in Sensei Tips.)

Process Step: A number assigned for each step in the process for future reference.
Process Name: A short name to describe the process.

Type: An organizational descriptor for each process step (i.e., database, Excel spreadsheet reference, EMR screen, email, wait for signature, link, etc.).

Begin Time: The time when the process step starts.

Operation (or Cycle) Time: The actual time for the process step to be completed. This should equal the difference between the Begin Time and the End Time.

End Time: The time when the process step stops.

Value-Added or Value-Enabled?: The categorization of the step as Value-Added or Value-Enabled (Yes) or Non Value-Added (No).

Value-Added Total: The cumulative Value-Added Time. Valued-Added is what the customer is willing to pay for.

Value-Enabled are the non-essential steps but are considered mandatory from a regulatory standpoint.

3. Color-code the various categories (e.g., green for VA, red for NVA, etc.) for more visual impact, and to facilitate ease of analysis.

4. Collect data for each of the process steps.

5. Create a table or chart to display the Value-Added Total time relative to the Non Value-Added Total time, as well as any other significant categories that may shed more light onto the problem or issue being investigated.

Further visualization of the data using the Chart Wizard in Excel will help you "see" data as pertinent information.

6. Brainstorm with the team to eliminate the Non Valued-Added activities or steps, minimize the Value-Enabled activities or steps, and maximize the Value-Added activities or steps.

The following benefits can be obtained by using the VA versus NVA Analysis:

❖ Help to determine slowest process or bottleneck within a value stream

❖ Allow process data to be analyzed with actual times

❖ Bring attention to the activities within the process being analyzed

❖ Ensure consensus on needed improvements when NVA time is significant

---

Sensei Tips for VA versus NVA Analysis

The following is an example of a VA versus NVA Analysis:

Value-Added versus Non Value-Added Analysis

Name of Team:
New Patient Experience Improvement Team

Shaded or green color signifies value-added and value-enabled times.

VA versus NVA Objective: Document the various start and stop times for the activities that comprise the process or value stream map.

Shaded or red color signifies possible non value-added time.

Date:
June 5

Shaded or yellow color signifies begin and end times for the activity.

Process Step	Process Name (Definition of Step)	Type	Begin Time	Operation Time	End Time	Value-Added or Value-Enabled?	Value-Added Total
1	Sign-In	Process	0:00:00	0:00:25	0:00:25	No	0:00:00
2	Ask and photocopy patient insurance information	Process	0:00:25	0:01:30	0:01:55	Yes	0:01:30
3	Ask and photocopy patient Driver's License	Process	0:01:55	0:01:30	0:02:25	Yes	0:03:00
4	Provide new patient paperwork and HIPAA consent forms	Process	0:02:25	0:00:10	0:02:35	Yes	0:03:10
5	Patient sits and completes paperwork	Process	0:02:35	0:15:00	0:17:35	Yes	0:18:10
6	Patient takes completed paperwork to front desk	Transport	0:17:35	0:00:30	0:18:05	Yes	0:18:40
7	Patient sits	Delay	0:18:05	0:20:00	0:38:05	No	0:18:40
8	Review all paperwork	Decision	0:38:05	0:02:00	0:40:05	Yes	0:20:40
9	Scan paperwork into EMR	Process	0:40:05	0:01:00	0:41:05	Yes	0:21:40
10	Patient gets called back to nurse's station	Transport	0:41:05	0:01:00	0:42:05	Yes	0:22:40
11	Height, weight	Process	0:42:05	0:01:30	0:43:35	Yes	0:24:10
12	Walk to exam room	Transport	0:43:35	0:00:30	0:44:05	Yes	0:24:40
13	H&P, BP, temp, and CC	Process	0:44:05	0:02:00	0:46:05	Yes	0:26:40
14	Patient waits	Delay	0:46:05	0:05:00	0:51:05	No	0:26:40
15	Doc enters room	End	0:51:05	End	End	End	End

The above analysis shows that there are opportunities for improvement given that there is nearly 50% of non value-added time associated with new patient visits. The analysis shows that it takes roughly 51 minutes for the patient to see a provider (i.e., process steps 1 - 15). While brainstorming different ways to minimize non value-added time, the team recommended and subsequently implemented a Web portal for new patients to complete their patient paperwork (i.e., process steps 4 - 6) prior to the visit. The new patient information is pulled directly into their registration software and EMR. Initial results were very favorable for the patient experience; new patients who completed paperwork prior to their visit had their wait times reduced by 38%. Within 1 year, 80% of all new patients were using the Web portal. This change, along with other improvements, allowed the practice to add additional appointments to the schedule without adding staff. By removing these steps and having the patient information directly entered into the software system, data entry errors were practically eliminated.

Constraint or Bottleneck Analysis

Give me six hours to chop down a tree and I will spend the first four sharpening the axe.
Abraham Lincoln

What is it?

A **Constraint or Bottleneck Analysis** is the identification of the slowest process step(s) in the product or service being provided. It can be done in a number of ways and is commonly called the constraint or bottleneck of a process. If a VA versus NVA Analysis (previous section) has been completed, the constraint is simply the slowest process step in the sequence. Consider additional reading on Theory of Constraints.

What does it do?

A constraint or bottleneck will usually lead to a backup, delay, or added wait time. Applying a thorough analysis with subsequent improvements can help alleviate many of these constraints. For example, turnaround times in the OR, bed availability, improving LWBS in the ED, getting patients discharged, etc. all have potential bottlenecks or constraints that impede work/patient flow, and therefore services. Applying a thorough analysis with subsequent improvements can help alleviate many of these constraints.

How do you do it?

The following steps or guidelines are used to conduct a Constraint or Bottleneck Analysis:

1. Obtain the VA versus NVA Analysis data.

2. Create a Bar Chart representing the Process Step, Process Name, Operation (or Cycle) Time, and any other key attributes.

3. Review the Bar Chart and note 2 to 3 of the highest numbers.

4. Determine if the higher number processes are value-added or non value-added.

Constraint or Bottleneck Analysis   87

5. Brainstorm with the team and determine how the non value-added (or constraints) can be reduced or eliminated.

6. Continue to work on reducing other process cycle times that impede flow.

The following benefits can be obtained by conducting a constraint or bottleneck analysis:

- ❖ Assist to organize data sets
- ❖ Allow for the slowest process to be easily identified
- ❖ Create opportunities for improvement
- ❖ Detail the entire process
- ❖ Bring attention to the "bottleneck" process steps relative to the entire process

Sensei Tips for Constraint or Bottleneck Analysis

The following is data from the previous Value-Added versus Non Value-Added Analysis table as a Bar Chart:

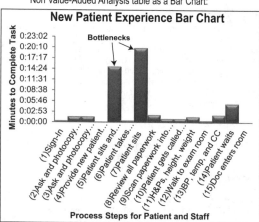

The Bar Chart of the data set from the Value-Added versus Non Value-Added Analysis on page 86 clearly shows the main constraints or bottlenecks. Additional charting can be done once the data set has been obtained.

Demand Analysis Plots and Takt Time

*If what you're working for really matters,
you'll give it all you've got.*
Nido Quebin

What is it?

Demand Analysis Plots are used to understand the pace of customer demand. Takt Time is the rate that a product or service needs to be completed in order to meet a customer demand. Understanding the pace of demand is critical to implementing improvement activities. The two primary methods for illustrating and calculating customer demand are Demand Analysis Plots and Takt Time.

What does it do?

Takt Time

Takt time defines the pace of repetitive customer demand. Takt time is presented in units of time and is calculated with the following equation:

Takt Time = Time available to work / Average daily demand

The available work time is the total available work time minus time for meetings, breaks, and any other non value-added activities and/or any time that the process is not available.

For example, the takt time for lab blood draws for ICU patients are:

Available hours of operation (Time available to work)

	Shifts: 1 @ 8 hours =	480 minutes
(-)	Breaks: 2 @ 15 minutes per =	30 minutes
	Available time to work =	450 minutes

	Lab orders ICU patients for 3 months =	1500
(/)	Working days 20 per month =	60
	Average daily demand (or blood draws) =	25

Takt time = 450 minutes / 25 blood draws = 18 minute takt time

Measure

This 18 minute takt time is the time the lab has to provide the service. Takt time for this value stream (i.e., ICU patients blood draws) must be balanced with the requirements of other value streams (e.g., clinics, pediatrics, floors, etc.) to ensure people, equipment, and resources are scheduled appropriately.

Takt time accomplishes the following:

- ❖ Align internal work rate to customer (or patient) demand rate - similar to a metronome keeping pace for playing a musical instrument or a drill sergeant calling out the "cadence" to ensure everyone marches in order
- ❖ Focus awareness on the customer
- ❖ Set a standard rate for all staff to meet and be measured against

Demand Analysis Plots

Demand Analysis Plots identify customer demand in terms of transactions or needs over a given time period for more non-repetitive goods or services. The historical or proposed current demand is plotted relative to a time period (i.e., one day, to one year, or season) or another variable depending on the type of good or service provided. In healthcare, demand analysis plots are very common and are used to staff areas appropriately. This is very helpful due to the perceived unpredictability of the flow of the patient.

By conducting a current demand analysis, some of the following actions may be implemented to improve the patient experience:

- ❖ Predictive scheduling - allocating resources over time given the historical records to level the work load throughout the day
- ❖ Stagger/start times for certain procedures/services
- ❖ Swing shifts for staff
- ❖ Part-time employees
- ❖ Volunteers assisting in various capacities

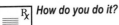

How do you do it?

The following steps or guidelines are used to create a Demand Analysis Plot and/or determine takt time:

1. Obtain data on customer demand.

2. If demand is repetitive, use the takt time formula.

3. If demand is non-repetitive, use a Demand Analysis Plot.

4. Use data from (2) and (3) and allocate resources accordingly.

Note: There may be times when segments of the Demand Analysis Plot will be used to calculate a takt time (for that specific period). The overall goal is to ensure resources are available to meet customer demand while ensuring no waste occurs.

The following benefits can be obtained by using Demand Analysis Plots or takt time:

- ❖ Quantify customer demand
- ❖ Allow resources to be adequately scheduled
- ❖ Reduce employee stress
- ❖ Ensure customer demand is met
- ❖ Minimize waste of overprocessing (i.e., over scheduling) and delay
- ❖ Improve customer satisfaction

Measure

Sensei Tips for Demand Analysis Plots and Takt Time

The following are examples of a Demand Analysis Plot and Takt Time:

Takt Time Example

An ED improvement team wants to use takt time to determine the demand for ED. The following are their calculations:

Time: 1440 minutes (60 minutes x 24 hours)
Volume: 1575 patients in 15 days by shifts (60 + 135 + 255 + 390 + 480 + 255)
Volume for 1 day (average): 1575 / 15 = 105 patients per 24 hour period
Takt time: 1440 minutes / 105 patients = 13.7 or approximately 14 minutes

However, this did not seem practical to work to this particular takt time and the team subsequently calculated takt time in 4 hour increments. The team was surprised to see that the takt time varied so much in each block of time. They knew that the ED was busier on the evening shift, but there was clearly a big difference between 0000 to 0400, and 1600 to 2000. "We need to change our staffing levels in ED," said one of the team members. But the Lean Sensei quickly said, "Don't jump to solutions yet! We have a lot more Lean tools to consider before we make any changes." For example, it may be necessary to correlate the patient acuity level with the actual skilled resources required for delivering patient care within each time increment. The team realized calculating takt time is just one aspect to solving a problem or initiating an improvement.

Takt Times for ED

Hours	Available Time (minutes) (4 hours x 60 minutes)	Patient Volume (Average per 4 hours)	Takt Time (Time/Volume)
0000 - 0400	240	4	60
0400 - 0800	240	9	27
0800 - 1200	240	17	14
1200 - 1600	240	26	9
1600 - 2000	240	32	8
2000 - 2400	240	17	14

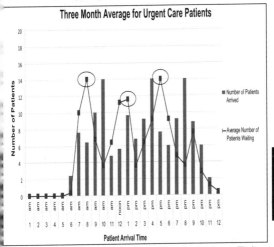

Three Month Average for Urgent Care Patients

Legend:
- Number of Patients Arrived
- Average Number of Patients Waiting

Y-axis: Number of Patients

X-axis: Patient Arrival Time

This Urgent Care Clinic is open from 6:00 am to 12:00 pm. Their Demand Analysis Plot clearly shows a backlog of patients at three different times throughout the day for Average Number of Patients Waiting (8:00 am, 1:00 pm, and 5:00 pm). The improvement team used this initial analysis, along with creating two process flowcharts, and subsequently streamlined the Triage process as well as the PA's time. Within 2 months the Average Number of Patients Waiting was reduced by 38%.

Measure

Voice of the Customer (VOC)

*Revolve your world around the customer and more
customers will revolve around you.*
Heather Williams

What is it?

Voice of the Customer (VOC) is a term used in business and Information Technology to describe the in-depth process of capturing a customer's expectations, preferences, and aversions. The VOC tool is a process that will deliver a greater understanding of a customer's expressed and unexpressed needs. The VOC is done by conducting market research through a variety of potential methods. Customer needs then can be ranked and prioritized to create an improved process. A common tool to do this is the customer feedback survey. Other tools intended to create a better understanding of customer desires are: focus group studies, complaint analysis, internet monitoring, and customer interviews. In each case, customer needs and priorities are documented and used for further analysis.

What does it do?

The VOC is also used today to maximize positive quality attributes (i.e., convenience, ease-to-do-business with, etc.). This creates value for the customer which leads to customer satisfaction and loyalty. *Just because an organization is doing nothing wrong does not mean they are doing everything right!*

The objectives of the VOC tool or process are to develop specific and measurable needs or specifications, provide a common language for the improvement team and provide input for new and innovative products and services. There are basically five levels of activities in the VOC process. Teams must decide which levels will provide the best fit for the scope and duration of the project. The five levels are:

1. *Relationship tracking* - This is used when organizations need to track the quality of customer relationships over time.

2. *Interaction monitoring* - This is used when every customer interaction, from a web-based or online transaction to a phone call, is important. Organizations need a way to monitor how effectively they handle these.

1. *Continuous listening* - This is used when you need to hear what customers are saying, such as listening to phone calls, reading blogs, reading inbound emails, and visiting appropriate customer locations.

2. *Project infusion* - This is used when new services need to be provided and insights about customers are needed. Despite the clear need for this type of effort, many organizations lack a formalized approach.

3. *Periodic immersion* - This is used when employees need to understand the product and services that are being offered, but from the customer's perspective. This involves spending a significant amount of time interacting directly with customers.

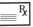

How do you do it?

The following steps or guidelines are used to create a Voice of the Customer survey:

1. Create a multi-disciplinary team.

2. Analyze current customer satisfaction levels.

3. Determine competitor's strengths and weaknesses as well as yours.

4. Use quantitative (i.e., complaint logs, etc.) and qualitative methods (Press-Ganey, patient evals, etc.) to determine survey questions.

5. Address the quality of the questions, legitimacy and accuracy of the data, as well as how useful the information is.

6. Use a representative sample of the customer base to gather the data.

7. Analyze the data for input by creating a Quality Function Deployment analysis (next section).

The following benefits can be obtained by conducting a Voice of the Customer survey:

- ❖ Develop specific and measurable needs of the customer
- ❖ Provide a common language for the improvement team
- ❖ Provide input for new and innovative products and/or services

Sensei Tips for Voice of the Customer

The following VOC was used to include areas outside the specific Dispo-to-Admit value stream to further understand the entire ED value stream. This information is then part of a Quality Function Deployment (next section).

Voice of the Customer (VOC) ED/Inpt Survey

In an effort to improve our Emergency Room services we are requesting you fill out this survey. Focus your attention to the timeframe between being notified of being admitted to the time of bed placement.

PLEASE SEND THIS WITH YOUR DINNER MENU SELECTION TODAY!

Name:_____ Date:_____

1. Of the following options, what is most important to providing you with the best ER experience possible?
   Rank 1 - 5 in order of importance with 1 being the most important and 5 the least important.

   _____ Skill of physicians/nurses   _____ Cleanliness

   _____ Attitude of staff   _____ Timeliness/waiting

   _____ Keeping me informed of care plan   _____ Keeping me informed of delays

2. Please estimate the time and service levels you experienced from the time you received the information you were to be admitted to the time you were in the hospital bed.

	How long? Note minutes or hours.	Was this acceptable?	If No, how long would have been acceptable? Note minutes or hours.
From the time you were told you would be admitted, to the time you were told that you were definitely going to be admitted?		Yes No	
From the time you were told you were going to be admitted, until you (or your family) were told your room number?		Yes No	
From the time you knew what unit and/or room number you would be going to, until the time you left the ED?		Yes No	
From the time you left the ED, until the time you were comfortably positioned in your inpatient bed?		Yes No	

3. Would you choose one hospital for ER care over another if you knew that a doctor would see you within 30 minutes?
   Circle one.   Yes   No

4. Is there anything else that you would like us to know, either good or bad, about your ER visit?

Thank you very much for your time in completing this survey. This information will be very helpful in improving the service we provide to you (and your family).

Note: Nearly 80% of companies currently use email for collecting customer feedback, but only 22% use social media sites and only 3% use iPhone applications.

Quality Function Deployment (QFD)

Quality is remembered long after the price is forgotten.
Gucci Family

What is it?

Quality Function Deployment (QFD) *is a tool that takes the VOC information and turns it into specific and measurable quality requirements that can be used to design improved service processes.* QFD methods provide a systematic approach to the design of a quality process. For example, QFD takes the VOC statement such as "We had to wait over 45 minutes to see the doctor, even though we had an appointment." to "All patients will be seen within 15 minutes."

What does it do?

QFD uses a comprehensive matrix system to relate VOC priorities to specific measurable characteristics and to a quality measurement and improvement plan.

Ensure the amount of information in the matrix is at a manageable level. A more complex QFD (or House of Quality) can include degrees of interaction and strength of relationship between the Customer Requirements, Organizational Requirements, and Technical Requirements. If this is your first QFD, it is recommended to keep it as simple as possible!

Measure

| R̲x̲ | ### How do you do it?

The following steps or guidelines can be used to create a Quality Function Deployment matrix:

1. Identify Customer Requirements and then determine the Customer Priority ratings for those requirements. This information would be derived from the VOC survey (or similar-type instrument). Address the unspoken needs (assumed and excitement capabilities), if appropriate.

2. List current Organizational Requirements which may include competitive pressures.

3. List Technical (and Procedural) Requirements.

4. Construct the basic QFD diagram and populate it with the appropriate data (information from 1 - 3).

5. Identify on the QFD diagram where the Organizational (O) and Technical Requirements (X) impact each Customer Requirement by placing an O or X in the corresponding box. This process is expected to create dialog and learning, as well as an updated QFD. An overlap is indicated on the QFD with an O and X - "⊗" symbol. These are strong relationships and are critical areas to address and improve. Be sparing with the strong relationship symbol.

6. Determine improvement initiatives to close the gaps. Assess whether the difficult items can be accomplished within the current project budget and schedule.

The following are the benefits that can be obtained by using a Quality Function Deployment matrix:

❖ Allow the VOC survey results to be quantified
❖ Focus improvements on customer requirements
❖ Leverage organizational and technical strengths to customer needs (and vice versa)
❖ Align business resources to key customer requirements

Sensei Tips for Quality Function Deployment

The following is an example of the Quality Function Deployment tool:

QFD Dispo to Inpt Bed Arrival	1	2	3	4	5	6	7	8		
Customer Priority / **Customer Requirements (Voice of the Customer)**	Organizational Requirements (O) / Staffing	Safety	HIPPA	Cost	Protocols	Communications	Bed Management		Current Measures	Competitive Measures
1 Keep me informed of care at all times	X	⊗	X	⊗	X	X	X		88.6%	98-99.9%
2 Assign right bed, first time	X	X	O		X	X	X		92.9%	99-100%
3 Transport to bed in timely manner	⊗	O	X	O		O			77.9%	98-99.9%
4 Care teams effective in the transfer of care	O		⊗	X		X	X		95.0%	96-99.9%
Technical Requirements (X)	EMR Updates	MEDs	Orders	Pain Management	Meals	Belongings	Insurances			
	1	2	3	4	5	6	7	8		

This Quality Function Deployment tool example (data from the Voice of the Customer Survey in previous chapter's example) determined the impact of the Organizational and Technical Requirements of the organization. The team believes that both the Technical Requirements of "EMR Updates" and the Organizational Requirements of "Staffing" can potentially impact the Customer Requirements of "Transport (patient) to bed in timely manner." This dual relationship is shown by placing both an "O" (Organizational Requirements) and an "X" (Technical Requirements) in the corresponding box. This dual marking is shown by a "⊗." The impact and relationships decisions are usually agreed through discussion by the team before moving on.

Measure

Measurement System Analysis (MSA)

What gets measured gets done, what gets measured properly, gets done properly.

Anonymous

What is it?

A **Measurement System Analysis (MSA)** *is a specially designed experiment that seeks to identify the components of variation in the measurement system.* Often measurements are made with little regard for the quality (accuracy) of such measurements. All too often, the measurements are not representative of the true value of the characteristic being measured. This might be because the measurement system is not accurate or precise enough which introduces bias into the measurement, or is not being used by properly by the staff.

What does it do?

Measurement System Analysis evaluates the test method, measuring instruments, and the entire process of obtaining measurements to ensure the integrity of data used for analysis and to understand the implications of measurement error for decisions made about a product or process. MSA is an important element of Six Sigma methodology and of other quality management systems.

Anytime something is measured (e.g., fluids, specifications-to-standards, staff satisfaction, etc.) there are actually two types of variation:

1. The variation within the process being examined (P)
2. The variation within the measurement system itself (M)

The total variation being examined (T) can be explained by a formula:

$$T = P + M$$

In a perfect world, the variation due to M (measurement system) would be zero, meaning that the only variation observed would be due to the process (P). In reality, there is often enough variation with the measurement system that true variation of the process cannot be defined. This is especially so in qualitative surveys. If this is the case, an improvement team's efforts to improve the process may only lead to frustration, as the measurement system masked the true variation of the process.

This is why MSA is so important. Improvement teams should complete MSAs to determine what portion of the total variation is due to the process and how much is due to the actual measurement system.

MSA analyzes the measurement system error to equipment, operations, procedures, software, and personnel. MSA is a critical first step that should precede any data-based decision-making, including SPC, Correlation and Regression Analysis, and Design of Experiments.

A Measurement System Analysis considers the following:

- ❖ Select the correct measurement and approach
- ❖ Assess the measuring device or instrument
- ❖ Assess procedures and employees
- ❖ Assess any measurement interactions
- ❖ Calculate the measurement uncertainty of individual measurement devices and/or measurement systems

Following are general requirements of all capable measurement systems:

- ❖ Statistically is stable over time (process is in control)
- ❖ Variability is small compared to the process variability
- ❖ Variability is small compared to the specification limits (tolerance)
- ❖ The resolution, or discrimination, of the measurement device must be small relative to the smaller of either the specification tolerance or the process spread (variation). As a rule of thumb, the measurement system should have resolution of at least 1/10th the smaller of either the specification tolerance or the process spread. If the resolution is not fine enough, process variability will not be recognized by the measurement system, thus blunting its effectiveness.

A measurement system can be characterized, or described, in the following five ways:

Accuracy or Location (Average Measurement Value vs. Actual Value)

1. Stability refers to the capacity of a measurement system to produce the same values over time when measuring the same sample. As with Statistical Process Control charts, stability means the absence of "Special Cause Variation," leaving only "Common Cause Variation" (random variation).

2. Bias, sometimes referred to as Accuracy, is a measure of the distance between the average value of the measurements and the "True" or "Actual" value of the sample or part. (See the illustration below.)

3. Linearity is a measure of the consistency of Bias over the range of the measurement device. For example, if a bathroom scale is under by 1.0 pound when measuring a 150 pound person, but is off by 5.0 pounds when measuring a 200 pound person, the scale Bias is non-linear in the sense that the degree of Bias changes over the range of use.

Precision or Variation (Spread of Measurement Values)

4. Repeatability assesses whether the *same* appraiser can measure the same part/sample/process multiple times with the same measurement device and get the same value.

5. Reproducibility assesses whether *different* appraisers can measure the same part/sample/process with the same measurement device and get the same value.

The diagram below illustrates the difference between the terms "Accuracy" and "Precision:"

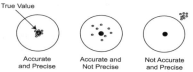

True Value

Accurate and Precise   Accurate and Not Precise   Not Accurate and Precise   Not Accurate and Not Precise

Efforts to improve measurement system quality are aimed at improving both accuracy and precision.

Factors affecting measurement systems might include:

- ❖ Equipment: measuring instrument, calibration, fixturing, etc.
- ❖ People: staff, training, education, skill level, etc.
- ❖ Process: test method, specification
- ❖ Samples: materials, items to be tested (sometimes called "parts"), sampling plan, sample preparation, process, etc.
- ❖ Environment: temperature, humidity, conditioning, pre-conditioning (i.e., interview or question bias), etc.
- ❖ Management: training programs, metrology system, support of people, support of quality management system, etc.

These can be plotted in a Cause and Effect or "Fishbone" Diagram (discussed in the Analyze Phase) to help identify potential sources of measurement variation.

Common tools and techniques of Measurement System Analysis include:

- ❖ Calibration studies
- ❖ Fixed effect ANOVA
- ❖ ANOVA Gage R&R
- ❖ Destructive Testing Analysis, and others
- ❖ Attribute Gage Study
- ❖ Components of variance
- ❖ Gage R&R

The tool selected is usually determined by characteristics of the measurement system itself. (Further study is needed beyond the scope of this book on many of these tools.) Two basic types of MSA tools are the Gage R & R study and the Attribute Gage study.

Gage R & R study is used when dealing with variable data (data we can measure like weight, distance, etc.). This stands for Gage Repeatability & Reproducibility.

Attribute Gage study is used when dealing with attribute data (pass/fail, good/bad, etc.).

When using a new measurement system for a characteristic which has not been previously measured on it, a measurement capability analysis should be performed. Measurement capability analyses are critical to the success of every measurement and ensure that future measurements will be representative of the process characteristic being measured.

How do you do it?

The following six rules are fundamental to performing a meaningful study and will help organizations perform a good gage capability studies.

1. Measurements or observations, if applicable, should be made in a random order to ensure that any drift or changes that occur due to unknown factors will be spread randomly throughout the study.

2. The worker or process should be unaware of what is being measured in order to avoid any possible knowledge bias. However, the person conducting the study (i.e., the observer) should be familiar with the process and record the data accordingly.

Measure

3. The readings should be estimated to the nearest number (use seconds or minutes) that can be obtained using identical instruments.

4. The study should be observed by a person who recognizes the importance of the caution required in conducting a reliable study.

5. The measurement procedure should be documented and all observers trained to the procedure prior to the study.

6. Each observer should use the same procedure to obtain the readings.

The following benefits can be obtained by implementing the MSA system:

- ❖ Allow for the correct measurement and approach
- ❖ Assess the measuring device
- ❖ Assess measurement interactions
- ❖ Help to define measurement uncertainties

 Sensei Tips for Measurement System Analysis

This following refers to the data collection Gage R&R on page 105 and references the Value-Added versus Non Value-Added Analysis on page 86:

1. The long method Gage R&R (GRR) study was used to validate the MSA.
2. Two observers (Don and Mary) observed 10 steps from the new patient experience from the time the patient signed-in until the Provider entered the exam room.
3. Findings (measurement of X's) were recorded on the data collection tool at the same time using the Process Name (Definition of Step) column (page 86) as a guide.
4. A new patient was randomly selected to follow through the process.
5. Data from the two samples determined the measurement error using the average range: (GRR=5.15(R/d).
6. The measurement percent of tolerance (GRR/tolerance) X 100 was determined. (If the Gage R&R is >20% you need redefine the Definition of Steps, reeducate the assessors, and then conduct the assessment again. If the Gage R&R is <20, then you can move forward with confidence and collect the data given the Definition of Steps.)
7. The measurement system was determined to be acceptable.

Process Steps	Observer (1) Don New Pt Smith	Observer (2) Mary New Pt Smith	Range	
	GRR SHORT METHOD (10 Observations)			
1	24	24	0	
2	92	93	1	
3	88	89	1	
4	8	10	2	
5	907	906	1	
6	32	32	0	
7	1188	1190	2	
8	124	123	1	
9	58	58	0	
10	62	62	0	
			8	Sum
			0.8	Average Range
			1.16	d
			0.69	Stdev(msr)
			3.55	GRR=5.15*stdev(msr)
			20	Tolerance
			18%	GRR % tolerance = GRR/Tolerance
			169239.32	Var process
INPUTS			0%	GRR % Contribution = var(msr)/var(total) * 100

A MSA was conducted to validate the data collection method to identify opportunities for improvement with the deployment of a Web-based new patient portal application. As part of the MSA, a Gage R&R was used to validate the data collection method. The example shown above is from the Process Steps 1 - 10 on page 86 of the Value-Added versus Non Value-Added Analysis. This data needs to be collected on new patients. The data cannot be collected for one day; therefore to get sample of patients across the spectrum, other observers needed to be trained. This was done using the Gage R&R that determines whether method in which the data is collected is reliable and repeatable. This example shows two observers (Don and Mary) who followed the same patient through their visit (first 10 steps). Observers 1 and 2 were within the acceptable of less than 20% of 0% [GRR % Contribution = var(msr)/var(total) * 100] tolerance which demonstrates the assessment tool was reliable and repeatable.

In Phase 1, prior to their appointment, new patients were sent the forms and were asked to bring them completed when they came for their appointment. In Phase II, a secured Web portal allowed patients to log-in so they could complete their paper work in the Electronic Medical Record (EMR) system prior to the appointment. This information was then pulled from the scheduling system into their EMR system. This reduced the overall wait time by 38% for new patient visits. Phase III was the roll-out for all patients prior to their visits to create a log-in and ID and ensure their personal and insurance information was up-to-date.

Process Capability

The best way to escape from a problem is to sovle it.
Alan Saporta

What is it?

Process Capability analysis is used to determine if a process, given its natural process variation in a stable state, is capable of meeting customer specifications or requirements. Determining process stability is done by monitoring a process output over time, using Run Charts and/or Statistical Process Control. True improvement in a process is achieved by balancing stability with the capability of meeting customer requirements, otherwise known as process capability.

What does it do?

The definitions and formulas for process average, range, and standard deviation are used to estimate process capability and are as follows:

Process Average = Mean = X-Bar = Sum of all data points / Number of data points

Range = R = Difference between the largest and smallest data point

Standard Deviation (SD) = Root Mean Square (RMS) =
$$\sigma = [\text{Sum of } ((X - \text{X-bar})^2 / \text{Number of data points})]^{\frac{1}{2}}$$

Process capabilities are calculated as follows:

Cp = Process Capability = Tolerance Range / 6 σ

Cpu = Process capability to the upper tolerance limit = (Upper Tolerance Limit – Process Average) / 3 σ

Cpl = Process capability to the lower tolerance limit = (Process Average - Lower Tolerance limit) / 3 σ

Cpk = the lower of Cpu or Cpl = (Closest Specification Limit to Process Average – Process Average) / 3 σ

Estimates of long term process capability are best predicted by the Cpk value. Cpk considers both the process spread (σ) and the process centering to specification nominal. The standard deviation (SD) representing the process variation is proportional to the overall process spread. A process being 6σ or 6σ capable means that ± 6σ process width falls within the specifications or tolerance limits, as illustrated in the diagram below:

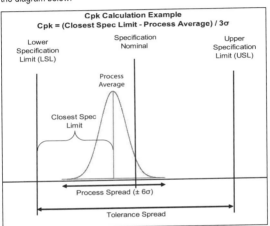

Cpk Calculation Example

Cpk = (Closest Spec Limit - Process Average) / 3σ

The following table shows the relationship between sigma level and Cpk (1.5 sigma long term shifts included):

Cpk	Sigma Level	Process Yield	PPM Defective
0.33	1	0.6827	691,462
0.67	2	0.9545	308,538
1	3	0.9973	66,807
1.33	4	0.9999	6,210
1.67	5	1	233
2	6	1	3.4

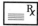 *How do you do it?*

The following steps or guidelines are used to determine and improve process capability:

1. Calculate from a data sample the process average and standard deviation using the formulas on page 106.

2. Determine the overall Process Capability (Cp) by dividing the total tolerance limit (Upper tolerance limit - Lower tolerance limit) by 6 SD's. This tells you the relationship of the width of the tolerance to the actual process output width, and if variation should be further reduced before moving forward. If the Cp is less than one, this means the process outputs are greater than the tolerance limits. If the Cp is 1.0 this means the process outputs are equal to the process tolerances, and if the Cp is greater than 1.0, this means that the actual process outputs are narrower than the process tolerances. The greater the Cp, the better.

3. Using the specification or tolerance limits, determine if the process average is closer to the upper or lower specification limit.

4. Using the closest specification limit to the actual process output average, take the difference between the process average and the closest specification limit, and divide it by 3 SD's. This is the Cpk which helps to determine if the process needs to be centered on the tolerance nominal, as well as a reduction of total variation.

5. Improve process capability by:
   a. Ensuring the process is centered on the specification nominal
   b. Reducing process output variation (which narrows the +/- 3 SD)
   c. Increasing the tolerance limits

The following benefits can be obtained by determining process capability:

- ❖ Allow for trends (problematic areas) to be easily viewed
- ❖ Reveal relationship between variables
- ❖ Identify whether the current process is capable of producing results within tolerance or customer needs
- ❖ Allow process owners to understand whether the process variation (SD), nominal (Average or X-bar), or both should be improved
- ❖ Reveal relationships between key process results such as average, SD, and tolerance limits
- ❖ Predict the success of the current process

Sensei Tips for Process Capability

The following is an example of process capability (from Minitab):

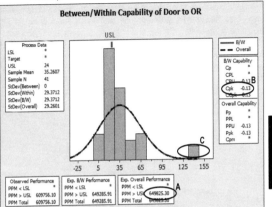

A high volume surgical center used Process Capability to analyze the performance of their current intake process for certain bone and joint fracture patients. This study focused on the cycle time of the patient experience from Emergency Room Quick Registration up to the patient entering the OR. The study's goal was to get the patient to the OR within 24 hours of arrival in the ER. Their analysis (chart above) showed the following: 649,825 (64.9%) (A) out of specification or defects or delayed transfers per million that means 351,175 ppm (34.1%) in specification or error free or on-time transfers per million of the patients either met or exceeded the goal of 24 hours. This produced a Cpk of less than 1 (i.e., -0.13) (B) which indicates the process in its current state is not capable of meeting the customer's specifications. The outlier (C) in the Histogram identifies a clear visual of an opportunity for improvement. The next steps to identify a solution for the outlier would be to map the entire process, introduce standard procedures, and load-level the work to insure that the center has the correct resources available at the right time to get the process started on time. The statistical analysis was very helpful in showing the process was not stable and provided the business case for process improvement.

Lean Thinking Statements for the Measure Phase

The following Lean Thinking Statement assessment should be done as an individual and, if desired, combined and discussed as a team. If the team leader realizes that many of the items are an issue for certain team members, then maybe a one-on-one with those specific individuals would be appropriate. Or, if a few of the team members have similar concerns over one or two of the statements, then possibly these should be addressed with the team. Continue with open and honest dialogue with the team. As a team member, it is YOUR responsibility to address any of the statements that hinder YOUR individual input to the team's progress. These statements are not to be taken lightly!

Use the 5 Level Likert Scale for the following statements:

> 1 - Strongly Disagree
> 2 - Disagree
> 3 - Neither Agree nor Disagree
> 4 - Agree
> 5 - Strongly Agree

I understand there are wastes in our processes. _____
I believe that the wastes can be either eliminate or minimized. _____
I understand our customer demands and requirements. _____
I believe we have a good, reliable measurement system. _____
I understand the difference between value-added and non value-added activities. _____
I can contribute to making our processes more capable. _____
I am confident in discussing this project with my colleagues. _____
I see the value in this team's approach. _____
I believe I can add value to this team. _____
I believe my ideas will be heard and considered. _____

Total Score: [   ]

If your score is less than 80% (40 points), then more work should be completed before moving on to the Analyze Phase. Ensure the A3 Project Report Section 3. Improvement Opportunity is nearly completed.

The Analyze Phase

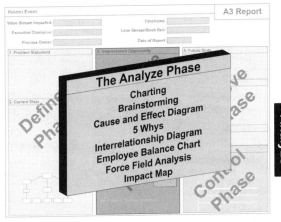

Tools listed in this section are most likely to be used at this time. All the tools can be applicable at any phase of a Kaizen Project as determined by the needs of the project team.

Charting

Begin with the end in mind.
Stephen Covey

What is it?

Charting is the process of making the most sense of the data. It is turning the "data" into useful information.

The **Pareto Chart** uses a bar chart format and represents the Pareto principle which states that 20% of the sources cause 80% of the problems.

The **Paynter Chart** is a visual representation over time relative to the subgroups based on Pareto Chart information. It is a further analysis of the bars of the Pareto Chart.

A **Pie Chart** is a circular chart divided into sectors, with each sector showing the relative size of each value. Pie Charts and Pareto Charts illustrate the same data. Pie Charts are typically used to compare multiple sets of data, where comparing the size of one Pie Chart to another can illustrate a difference in size or magnitude of the situations.

Scatter (and Concentration) Plots are used to study the possible relationship between one variable and another. Through visual examination and additional mathematical analysis, problem solvers can determine relationships between variables.

A **Radar Chart**, also known as a Spider Chart or a Star Chart, because of its appearance, plots the values of each category along a separate axis that starts in the center of the chart and ends on the outer ring.

A **Run Chart** is a method to display several data points over time. Because our minds are not good at remembering patterns in data, a visual display allows us to see the measurement(s) of an entire process.

Histograms utilize data and display the spread and shape of the distribution. Histograms are simple bar chart representations of the range, amount, and pattern of variation for data (i.e., the population).

Note: In Microsoft Office, the Chart Wizard can assist in creating many other types of charts within a few mouse clicks. Also, if more advanced data analysis is required, consider the Pivot Table function.

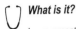

What is it?

Improvement teams more fully understand problems as they analyze data with a chart. Charts often become an impetus for improvement ideas. These charts help to prioritize and break down complex problems into smaller chunks. They also help to identify multiple root causes.

How do you do it?

The following steps or guidelines are used to assist in determining the type or types of charts to be used:

1. Gather a representative sample of data.

2. Review and create an appropriate chart by reviewing the following sample charts and their main attributes:

Pareto Chart

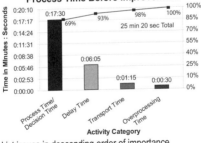

❖ List issues in descending order of importance
❖ Generally, tallest bars indicate biggest contributors to the problem
❖ Good for displaying before and after improvement initiatives

Paynter Chart

Paynter Chart of X-Ray Process Before Improvement

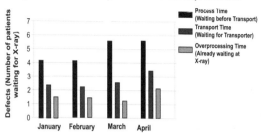

- ❖ Used to track defects over time relative to corrective action
- ❖ Similar to a Run Chart
- ❖ Paynter Chart goes beyond the Pareto by sub-grouping (or further categorizing) the Pareto bars which could be days, hours, etc.

Pie Chart

Pie Chart of X-Ray Process Time Before Improvement

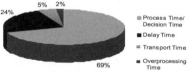

- ❖ Display relative size of each category to each other
- ❖ Good for comparing multiple sets of data, like changes that occur over time
- ❖ Illustrate a difference in size or magnitude of the data sets
- ❖ Allow for quick interpretation of the data

Scatter Plot

Actual to Estimated Equipment Purchase Cost

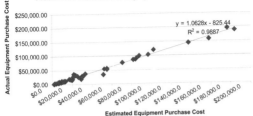

- ❖ Allow for trends (problematic areas) to be easily viewed
- ❖ Reveal relationship between variables
- ❖ Answer the question, are the variables related?
- ❖ Help to identify the "outliers" which may need further investigation
- ❖ Provide data for a linear regression if there is a high degree of positive or negative correlation
- ❖ Provide data for a non-linear regression if there is a small degree of positive or negative correlation

Radar Chart

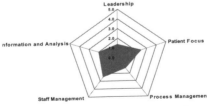

- ❖ Allow for a visual representation of the before and after measurements in one view
- ❖ Allow for multiple data sets to be compared to one another if colors or some other indicators are used
- ❖ Provide a visual to get a "feel" for data

Run Chart

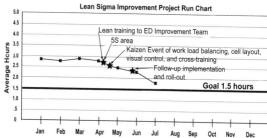

Lean Sigma Improvement Project Run Chart

- ❖ Allow improvements to be verified as effective
- ❖ Help to determine most effective long-term solutions
- ❖ Measure effectiveness of improvements
- ❖ Display improvement results over time

Histogram

Length of Stay Patients in a Hospital Unit in 1st week May

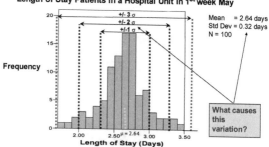

- ❖ Display data showing peaks and valleys, clusters, and outliers (i.e., data points numerically different from rest of the group)
- ❖ Allow visual representation of data sets
- ❖ Organize data into "bins" for additional analysis
- ❖ Typically, no fewer than 5 and no more than 20 class intervals or bins should be created. Histograms captures the shape of the distribution. Too few bins and the shape is lost. Too many bins and the shape is lost by the random fluctuations.

🍎 Sensei Tips for Charting

The following are examples of Charting:

Invasive Cardiology Value Stream: Data Collection Worksheet

Materials Needed:

1) 2 Sharpened Pencils with Eraser
2) Wrist Watch/Stopwatch (Must use same for all)
3) This Data Collection Worksheet

Patient MRN #: _____

Data Collector's Name: _____

Date: _____

Process Steps	Time (Military)	Operational Definition	Comments
Began Boarding Case	__ : __	Record time when CCL Systems Coordinator receives the call or fax to board an IC procedure.	
Finished Boarding Case	__ : __	Record time when CCL Systems Coordinator notifies Admitting.	
Record # of cases handed to Admitting at this time: _____			
Began Pre-Op Call	__ : __	Record time when Holding Room RN picks up phone to call patient for Hx.	
Finished Pre-Op Call	__ : __	Record time when Holding Room RN places paperwork in "Next Day" pile.	
Began Patient Arrival	__ : __	Record time when patient signs-in in Admitting.	
Finished Patient Arrival	__ : __	Record time when CCL associate picks up patient from Admitting.	

Good data collection techniques must be used before charting. This Data Collection Worksheet includes the operational definition of the categories to minimize confusion about what is to be measured.

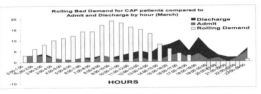

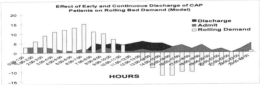

Examples of ER patient volume – see the differences between weekday average – top – and weekend average – bottom. Is the takt time the same? Be alert to changes in flow by hour, or by day – that's why measurement is so important. Base decisions on data!

Brainstorming

*A good plan is like a road map, it shows the final
destination and usually the best way to get there.*
H. Stanley Judd

What is it?

Brainstorming *is used to generate a high volume of ideas
with team members' full participation that is free of criticism
and judgment within a 5 - 15 minute time period.*

Note: In brainstorming, there is one cardinal rule:

No idea is criticized!

What does it do?

There are two basic methods of brainstorming: structured and
unstructured.

Structured - *A defined method in which each team member contributes
his/her ideas in order until all ideas are exhausted.* Use this if:

- ❖ The meeting has a dominate team member
- ❖ The unstructured approach has been used and numerous
  team members did not contribute their ideas
- ❖ Time is critical
- ❖ The facilitator is contributing too many of the ideas in an
  unstructured brainstorming method

Unstructured - *A method in which team members contribute their ideas
as they occur (or come to mind) until all ideas are exhausted.*

There are two methods to conduct an unstructured brainstorming
session:

Method 1: The facilitator documents any and all ideas from the team
members on a whiteboard or flip chart in no specific order or fashion.

Method 2: The facilitator provides Post-it Notes to each team member.
Each team member then writes their ideas on the Post-it Notes and
place them on the whiteboard, flip chart, or wall.

Note: Method 2 is preferred when some people find it difficult to speak in public. Allow a maximum of 15 minutes for either method.

How do you do it?

The following steps or guidelines are used to conduct a structured brainstorming session:

1. Find a quiet room with a flip chart or whiteboard (or have everyone log into the Remote Desktop Sharing or Web conferencing application at a particular time).

2. State the problem, gain a consensus, and write it down so everyone can see it. It is critical that everyone understand the issue or problem. The facilitator should get a visual or verbal confirmation from each team member that the problem is understood. Further clarification of the problem at this stage may lend insight to potential solutions. Do not rush this step!

3. Each team member provides an idea in a round robin fashion. Round robin is receiving one idea from each person in a circular manner until everyone has stated their idea. If a team member does not have an idea for their turn, then they can pass. This rotation process encourages full participation. It may also increase some team members' anxieties about having their ideas exposed. The facilitator should acknowledge this and be helpful to any person that seems shy.

4. The team facilitator or scribe documents each idea exactly how the person stated the idea, without any interpretation.

5. Collect the ideas until everyone has spoken, thus indicating all ideas are exhausted. This process should take 5 - 15 minutes, depending on how well the problem was stated.

6. Review the entire list once everyone has passed. Remove any ideas that are identical. If there are subtle differences keep them as separate ideas.

7. Show appreciation to everyone for their contributions.

Any type of brainstorming session starts with a clear question and ends with a raw list of ideas. Some ideas will be good and some will not. Once brainstorming is complete, duplicate (or similar type) ideas should be consolidated. Additional Lean Sigma tools and exercises will help to determine which of the ideas have the greatest impact on the identified problem.

Structured or unstructured brainstorming is used throughout any and all Lean Sigma projects, depending on the team's knowledge of the problem and the specific tools used. The principles of brainstorming are the same whether it is done in a conference room or through some type of Webinar or Web conferencing tool with the team members. For example, PersonalBrain101 is a Web-based program that allows you to add files, Web pages, integrate Outlook and Webmail, etc. via the Internet for sharing ideas. iBrainstorming is an iPad app that can be used. There are many other competitive applications that do similar functions.

The following benefits can be obtained by brainstorming:

- ❖ Allow all ideas to be explored
- ❖ Ensure input from all team members
- ❖ Encourage participation and consensus building

 Sensei Tips for Brainstorming

The following is an example of a two-person brainstorming session:

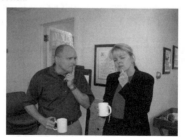

Brainstorming does not hurt (even though it seems these two team members are struggling)!

Cause and Effect (or Fishbone) Diagram

Life is a series of commas, not periods.
Matthew McConaughey

What is it?

Cause and Effect (or Fishbone) Diagrams allow a team to graphically display and explore, in increasing detail, all the possible causes of a problem or issue. This assists the team to determine the true root cause(s). The problem or effect is identified on the head of the diagram, and brainstorming and/or other data collection techniques are used to identify and prioritize all possible causes.

What does it do?

If done properly and completely, the cause(s) of the problem should be somewhere listed on the diagram. A Fishbone Diagram can be used once the problem (i.e., effect) has been clearly defined.

Be flexible in the major "bones" or "skeleton" categories that are used. Many times the main categories are Man, Method, Machine (Equipment, Information Technology, etc.), Material, and Mother Nature (Environmental Factors). There is no ideal set of categories or numbers. Make the categories relevant to your problem or improvement initiative.

How do you do it?

The following steps or guidelines are used to create a Fishbone Diagram:

1. Write the 4 - 6 main categories on a whiteboard, flip chart, or post/publish on a document sharing system.

2. Write the effect of the problem as the "head" of the fishbone.

3. List all possible causes of the problem (or effect) in the various 4 - 5 categories. Use brainstorming techniques to ensure all ideas are explored and documented on the Fishbone Diagram.

Cause and Effect (or Fishbone) Diagram

Analyze

4. Prioritize causes that need to be investigated further via data collection, beta test, etc.

5. Identify the top 1, 2, or 3 items.

6. Brainstorm with items selected in (5) through additional data collection or conduct a 5 Why Analysis (next section) on each item.

The following benefits can be obtained by creating a Fishbone Diagram:

❖ Define and displays the major causes, sub-causes, and root causes that are under investigation
❖ Provide a focus for a team for discussion and consensus building
❖ Visualize the possible relationships between causes
❖ Help to categorize potential causes into sub-groups

Sensei Tips for Cause and Effect (or Fishbone) Diagrams

The following is an example of a Fishbone Diagram:

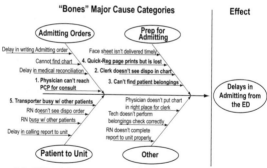

Numbered bold items are the main causes of Delays in Admitting from the ED (Emergency Department) via reaching a consensus from data collection methods.

This Emergency Department's Lean Sigma improvement team using the Fishbone Diagram created unique categories of Admitting Order, Prep for Admitting, Patient to Unit, and Other. These were the primary processes or "bones" that caused delays in admitting. The team further prioritized the top 5 potential reasons (noted by the numbered bold text).

5 Whys

It takes just as much energy to wish as it does to plan.
Eleanor Roosevelt

What is it?

5 Whys analysis allows organized brainstorming to methodically determine the causes of a problem (i.e., effect). Most often teams observe a symptom of the problem rather than the problem itself. Always ask "Why?" while arriving at the answer with data.

What does it do?

The 5 Whys is closely linked to the Fishbone (Cause and Effect) Diagram. The 5 Why analysis involves looking at a potential cause of a problem and asking: "Why?" and "What caused this problem?" as many times as it requires to get to the root cause. Very often, the answer to the first "why" will prompt another "why" and the answer to the second "why" will prompt another and so on; hence the name 5 Whys.

How do you do it?

The following steps or guidelines are used to conduct a 5 Why analysis:

1. List the top 2 - 5 potential main causes of the problem identified from the Fishbone Diagram. Use additional Pareto Charts to help identify or clarify the main potential causes, if appropriate.

2. Ask "Why" five times for each potential cause to get to the root cause.
   Note: Asking Why 5 times may or may not be required for each potential cause of the problem; the probable root cause may be identified after only 2 "Why?" questions.

3. Use the information and start a plan for additional data collection and testing or an improvement implementation activity.

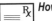

Analyze

Note: The 5 Why analysis can be done in a conference room or through a Webinar or Remote Desktop Sharing tool with the team members.

The following benefits can be obtained by conducting a 5 Why analysis:

- ❖ Help to quickly identify the root cause(s) of a problem
- ❖ Help to determine relationships between root causes
- ❖ Encourage participation and consensus building
- ❖ Adapt easily to all levels of the organization and is easy to use and understand

Note: The 5 Why analysis is data-driven (unlike brainstorming, which often is not).

 Sensei Tips for the 5 Whys

The following is an example of a 5 Why analysis:

5 Why Analysis				
Problem: Delay in patients being admitted from the ED to IP bed				
Cause 1. Physician can't reach PCP	**Cause 2. Clerk doesn't see dispo in chart**	**Cause 3. Patient belongings missing**	**Cause 4. Quick-Reg page gets lost**	**Cause 5. Transporter busy w/ other patients**
Why?	Why?	Why?	Why?	Why?
PCP doesn't answer page	Chart not given to clerk for filing	Belongings misplaced in Triage	No way to flag Quick-Reg page from others	Not enough transporters to handle calls quickly
Why?	Why?	Why?	Why?	Why?
PCP doesn't receive page	Doctor busy, doesn't want to walk to clerk	Hurry to get patient back to ED, no check	Can't color code, all pages the same	Budgeting/financial reasons
Why?	Why?	Why?	Why?	Why?
Wrong pager number	Doctor is focused on other patients	Focus on future, as more patients arrive	Not a vendor change programming option	Transporters considered non-direct care position
Why?	Why?	Why?	Why?	Why?
Information in computer listing not up-to-date	Doctor prefers to write notes			Transporters costs hit expenses directly; patient wait does not
Why?	Why?	Why?	Why?	Why?
No standard audit process to ensure info is up-to-date				

This 5 Why Analysis provided the team with 5 possible reasons for why there was a delay admitting patients from the ED. Note the potential root causes were on the 3rd, 4th, and 5th Whys.

Interrelationship Diagram

Pleasure in the job puts perfection in the work.
Aristotle

What is it?

*The **Interrelationship Diagram** is an analysis tool that allows a team to understand and identify the cause-and-effect relationships among critical issues.*

What does it do?

Interrelationship Diagrams are used to understand and illustrate the inputs, outputs, and relationships of key processes or data. They make it easy to identify the factors in a situation that drive the observed outcomes.

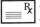

How do you do it?

The following steps or guidelines are used to create an Interrelationship Diagram:

1. Develop the problem or improvement statement and gain consensus among team members.

2. Develop issues around the problem or improvement statement (from brainstorming, 5 Why analysis, etc.). Write issues on Post-it Notes, if team is physically present.

3. Arrange the issues in a circular format.

4. Identify cause-and-effect relationships starting at any issue by determining if there is no cause/effect relationship, a weak cause/effect relationship, or a strong cause/effect relationship.

5. Draw arrows to indicate directions of influence. For each relationship pair identified in step 4, draw an arrow with solid lines to indicate strong relationships and an arrow with dashed lines to indicate weaker relationships. Always denote by the arrow in the direction of the strong issue. Never draw two-headed arrows.

6. Total the number of arrows going in and out for each issue.

7. Identify possible root cause(s) and process drivers from the problem or improvement statement noting the greater number of incoming arrows. Identify critical areas to improve that have the greatest impact on the problem or opportunity.

8. Use the information for proposed improvement activities.

The following benefits can be obtained by using the Interrelationship Diagram:

❖ Allow for understanding the links between ideas or cause-and-effect relationships
❖ Provide a process for analyzing complex issues

 Sensei Tips for Interrelationship Diagram

The following Interrelationship Diagram helps to determine the main factors for improving a physician group's patient experience:

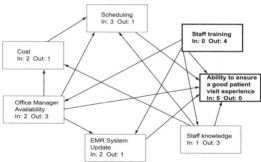

*The Interrelationship Diagram indicates that the most outputs (i.e., **Staff training In:0 Out:4**) is a key area for improvement as it affects the outcomes or results of many different areas. If this area is improved, the results or outcomes will improve many areas. The area with the most inputs (i.e., **Ability to ensure a good patient visit experience In:5 Out:0**) will be affected the most by any improvements implemented. For this example, it is clear that Staff training, with the large count of outgoing arrows, is the main driver of the process outcomes.*

Employee Balance Chart

Five frogs are sitting on a log. Four decide to jump
off. How many are left? Five. Because there's a
difference between deciding and doing.
Mark Feldman

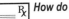 ### What is it?

The **Employee Balance Chart** is a visual display, in the form of a Bar Chart, that represents work elements and cycle times relative to the total value stream cycle time and takt time (or pitch). Create a current and future Employee Balance Chart.

What does it do?

The current state Employee Balance Chart analyzes the current state of how work relative to the value stream is allocated and ends with the future state Employee Balance Chart that represents an even and fair distribution of work. This ensures customer demand is met with a continuous flow mentality.

How do you do it?

The following steps or guidelines are used to create an Employee Balance Chart:

1. List processes from the current state value stream or process map on the horizontal axis of a graph. This is the current state Employee Balance Chart. Identify each process, its beginning and end, and any process parameters.

2. Obtain individual cycle times for each process step as well as the sub processes or tasks. Ensure times are accurate and reflect current processes. If a value stream map was created, each process total cycle time should match the process times located on the step graph at the bottom of the current state value stream map.

3. Calculate the takt time for the process or goal. Create a horizontal line to represent this time. The vertical axis scale should be 120% of the highest total single process cycle time.

4. Determine the ideal number of workers needed for a value stream, cell, or work area. When you determine the ideal number of workers to operate the process or processes for the value stream, keep in mind that the workers will most likely have multiple value streams they are responsible for throughout the day. The ideal number of workers is determined by dividing the total process cycle time by the takt time (or pitch). For example, in the lab, if an average blood draw takes 5 minutes (total cycle time) and the demand (takt time) is determined to be 5 minutes (12 patient draws per hour), the ideal number of workers needed will be 1 person (5 minutes total cycle time / 5 minute takt time). Use this to *assist* in determining staffing levels.

Note: If the decimal number from the takt time calculation is less than X.5 workers required, balance the value stream to the lesser whole number. Ensure each worker is balanced to takt time and allocate any excess time to one worker. Utilize the excess time to improve standard work procedures and conduct kaizen activities attempting to reduce additional wastes within the processes. Once the employee's efforts are no longer needed on the original project, that person can be placed in another continuous improvement capacity or position in the organization. Lean is not about reducing the number of people, it is about eliminating waste. Without this understanding, Lean will never be accepted. (Use the Standard Work Combination Table on page 169 to reduce process cycle times to meet takt time or goal.)

If the decimal number from the takt time calculation is equal to or greater than X.5, then balance to the larger whole number.

5. Brainstorm with the team and re-arrange processes or activities to ensure all process meet takt time or goals are met. This becomes the future state Employee Balance Chart.

6. Determine improvement activities to ensure step 5 is completed.

7. Create standard work procedures and train workers.

The future state Employee Balance Chart creates a clear, visual target. If there are difficulties reallocating work duties, or the takt time cannot be met within the current cycle times, consider Improve or Control Phase tools.

The following benefits can be obtained by creating an Employee Balance Chart:

- ❖ Assist to determine the number of workers needed for a given demand (or value stream)
- ❖ Allow for consensus for distributing (i.e., or represent) work units or activities
- ❖ Visualize cycle times for each process and sub-process
- ❖ Assist to standardize the process
- ❖ Improve productivity
- ❖ Promote the importance of cross-training

Sensei Tips for Employee Balance Chart

An improvement team for an Emergency Department created the following Current State Employee Balance Chart to assist in balancing the work load throughout the department:

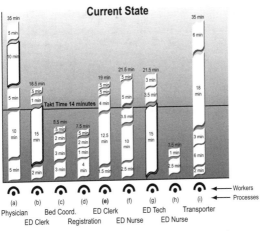

This Employee Balance Chart Current State indicates several process activities cannot meet the takt time of 14 minutes.

Analyze

The team brainstormed and displayed the following Lean Sigma tools on for their Future State Employee Balance Chart.

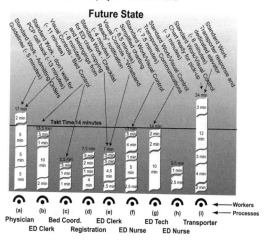

This Employee Balance Chart Future State displays the mini-Kaizens or PDCAs that need to be implemented. Even though all process activities could not be made to meet takt time, it is a good start.

Force Field Analysis

Never, never, never, never give up.
Sir Winston Churchill

What is it?

Force Field Analysis is an extremely useful tool for understanding and illustrating the forces for and against an idea, direction, decision, or strategy. The logic behind this technique is that when change occurs there are always two sides to change: one side is proactive and is driving the change while the other side is resistant to change and preventing change from occurring.

What does it do?

When using this technique, teams carefully identify, by means of a diagram, both the positive and negative forces and then find ways to enhance the forces that are pro-change and reduce the forces that resist change.

How do you do it?

The following steps or guidelines are used to conduct a Force Field Analysis:

1. Summarize the change and document it in a central location (i.e., someplace where comments can be listed for both sides).

2. Use brainstorming and list the forces driving the change.

3. Use brainstorming and list the forces resisting the change.

4. Estimate on a scale of 1 - 10 the estimated strength relative to the change.

5. Sum the strength ratings.

6. Use the information to better understand resistance to change in upcoming improvement activities.

Analyze

The following benefits can be obtained by conducting a Force Field Analysis:

❖ Allow everyone to participate
❖ Promote creative thought on proposed changes
❖ Assist to build consensus and gain process change buy-in
❖ Anticipate resistance systematically

 Sensei Tips for Force Field Analysis

The team created the following Force Field Analysis for an EMR upgrade:

Forces For Change	Forces Against Change
Patient information more quickly accessed	Already too busy
Ability to gather more data	Current system worked fine
Reduction in paperwork for staff and patients	Uncertainty and apprehension
Mandated by system and government	Disruption to current protocols
Proven successful	System bugs or failures
Accessible anytime	Training takes time and effort
Improve patient safety	

Impact Map

Even if you are on the right track, you will get run over if you just sit there.
Will Rogers

What is it?

The Impact Map allows teams to identify solutions most likely to have the greatest impact on the problem with the least effort. Opportunities and action ideas that have a high impact on the organization and are easily completed should take top implementation priority. Opportunities that have a high impact and take more time and effort to accomplish should be targeted next. Ideas that have little impact, but are easily completed should be done as time permits. Finally, projects or ideas that have a low potential impact on the organization and are difficult or expensive to implement could be considered at a later date. In summary, teams should reach a consensus on the EASE of implementation, as well as the IMPACT that it will have on the result.

What does it do?

Be sure the team does not spend too much time analyzing potential projects, as it is far more important to begin the improvement actions. Make sure the team always looks for low cost or no cost solutions first and advocates "creativity before capital" when considering action plans. Also, protect the customer and the organization by minimizing the risk of a proposed improvement not working. Ensure that the team can return the situation to the current state if the improvement idea fails.

Encourage teams to develop the Impact Map in a participative manner so everyone has the opportunity to express their thoughts and opinions. Dialogue and discussion are used to reach consensus on project priorities. Team members develop a high commitment and ownership to improvement activities only when they have an influence on projects. Impact Maps also provide an excellent communication vehicle for the improvement team.

Analyze

![Rx icon] **How do you do it?**

The following steps or guidelines are used to create an Impact Map:

1. List the proposed improvement activities or containment actions that are in place.

2. Create a graph with the vertical-axis denoting IMPACT: 1 is at the bottom (label as LOW) and 10 at the top (label as HIGH). Create the horizontal axis denoting EASE with the left as 1 (label as VERY EASY) and the far right as 10 (label as VERY DIFFICULT).

3. Divide the graph into four quadrants and label appropriately. See labels in Sensei Tips Impact Map example.

4. Brainstorm with the team and assign each item listed in step 1 to an area of the map.

5. Determine which items have the greatest impact with the least amount of effort. Consider these (and any others that may be practical to implement) as improvement activities.

6. Communicate to management those items that are very difficult and may have a high impact, but may be beyond the scope of this particular improvement project.

The following benefits can be obtained by creating an Impact Map:

❖ Help to prioritize improvement activities
❖ Provide an avenue to discuss improvement activities prior to implementation
❖ Allow for proposed improvement activities to be easily communicated to the organization

Sensei Tips for Impact Map

The team created the following Impact Map to prioritize improvement activities for the Dispo-to-Admit value stream:

	Impact Map		
	IMPACT of the result (1 - Very Low to 10 - Very High) EASE of achieving (1 - Very Easy to 10 - Very Difficult)		
No.	**Proposed Action Items**	**EASE**	**IMPACT**
1.	New standards for transporter communications	8	9
2.	Dedicate elevator for transporters	9	6
3.	Modify SOP for chart retrieval	8	10
4.	Update SOP for Admitting Orders Guidelines	4	3
5.	Create and communicate new bed control procedures	2	8
6.	Simplify and standardize new charting procedures	1	9
7.	Create new Wristband Ready notifications and train staff	8	7

```
       HIGH 10
            9   (6)              (3)
            8       Implement    (1)
                    Immediately  Develop
            7   (5)              Further
IMPACT                           (7)
            6
            5                    (2)
            4
            3   Develop Greater  Watch for
                Business Impact  Further
            2           (4)      Developments
            1
                1  2  3  4  5  6  7  8  9  10
                VERY            EASE          VERY
                EASY                          DIFFICULT
```

This Impact Map reveals that Items 5 and 6 will have the greatest impact and can be implemented immediately, while Items 1, 2, 3, 4, and 7 need either more data or further investigation before any implementation.

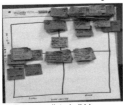

This team listed all ideas on Post-it Notes grouped around common themes.

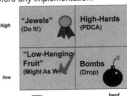

This team modified the Impact Map and used it to prioritized improvements.

Lean Thinking Statements for the Analyze Phase

The following Lean Thinking Statement assessment should be done as an individual and, if desired, combined and discussed as a team. If the team leader realizes that many of the items are an issue for certain team members, then maybe a one-on-one with those specific individuals would be appropriate. Or, if a few of the team members have similar concerns over one or two of the statements, then possibly these should be addressed with the team. Continue with open and honest dialogue with the team. As a team member, it is YOUR responsibility to address any of the statements that hinder YOUR individual input to the team's progress. These statements are not to be taken lightly!

Use the 5 Level Likert Scale for the following statements:

1 - Strongly Disagree
2 - Disagree
3 - Neither Agree nor Disagree
4 - Agree
5 - Strongly Agree

I understand the various charts that were created. _____
I contributed ideas in the brainstorming session. _____
I understand the value of using Employee Balance Charts. _____
I believe we had a good analysis on root causes and
solutions using Force Field Analysis and Impact Maps. _____
The Fishbone and 5 Why helped determine root cause. _____
I can contribute to this team. _____
I am confident in discussing this project with my colleagues. _____
I see the value in this team's approach. _____
I believe I can add value to this team. _____
I believe my ideas will be heard and considered. _____

Total Score: [　　]

If your score is less than 80% (40 points), then more work should be completed before moving on to the Improve Phase. Ensure the A3 Project Report Section 4. Problem Analysis is nearly completed.

Note: Charting will most likely also be used in the A3 Project Report Sections 7. Verify Results and 8. Follow-Up.

The Improve Phase

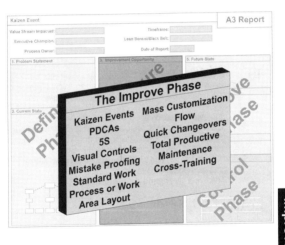

Kaizen Event | A3 Report
Value Stream Impacted: | Timeframe:
Executive Champion: | Lean Sensei/Black Belt:
Process Owner: | Date of Report:
1. Problem Statement | 3. Improvement Opportunity | 5. Future State
2. Current State

The Improve Phase

Kaizen Events
PDCAs
5S
Visual Controls
Mistake Proofing
Standard Work
Process or Work
Area Layout

Mass Customization
Flow
Quick Changeovers
Total Productive
Maintenance
Cross-Training

Improve

Tools listed in this section are most likely to be used at this time. All the tools can be applicable at any phase of a Kaizen Project as determined by the needs of the project team.

Kaizen Events

The problem is never how to get new, innovative thoughts into your mind, but how to get the old ones out.
    Dee Hock

What is it?

Kaizen Events, sometimes called "Rapid Improvement Events" or "Kaizen Blitzes" are targeted events conducted by improvement teams to implement improvements quickly in a specific area.

What does it do?

Teams use Kaizen Events to implement significant improvements in a relatively short time-frame. Use Kaizen Events instead of slower, incremental changes in the following circumstances:

❖   Improvement needs are urgent or at crisis levels.
❖   The area or process being addressed is continually in use by the organization and taking the area or process out of service can only be tolerated for a short while.
❖   Minimal training and facilitation can be afforded because of time or financial constraints.
❖   There is a very narrow area of focus.

How do you do it?

Kaizen Events are comprised of three parts:

Part 1. Planning Phase - all the activities to prepare the area or process for improvements
Part 2. PDCA Implementation Phase - all the activities to effectively implement process changes (i.e., improvements)
Part 3. Follow-Up Phase - all the activities to track and monitor to control improvements (for sustainability)

The PDCA Implementation Phase of a Kaizen Event can last anywhere from 1 - 2 hours to 3 - 5 days (depending on the scope of improvement).

The following are general guidelines for stakeholders of a Kaizen Event:

A. Management Actions (Planning Phase)
   1. Select an area, process, or product related to the Project Charter for rapid improvement.
   2. Create an initial Team Charter and process or value stream map.
   3. Assess opportunities and needs with current state measurement and analytical Lean Sigma tools.
   4. Establish short term improvement measures and goals.
   5. Select a Team Leader (who typically may be the process owner) and facilitator.
   6. Schedule dates with all stakeholders.

B. Team Leader Actions (Planning Phase)
   1. Determine and notify appropriate team members.
   2. Review Project and Team Charters.
   3. Create and distribute Meeting Agenda.
   4. Invite outside participants, if required.
   5. Conduct appropriate meetings prior to the dedicated days.

C. Team Leader and Team Actions (Planning Phase)
   1. Create or obtain current value stream or process map.
   2. Obtain current state or baseline measurements.
   3. Communicate and obtain alignment on objectives.
   4. Start a log of NVA activities (i.e., wastes) in the area.

D. Facilitator or Team Leader Actions (Planning Phase)
   1. Create work session detailed agendas and time lines.
   2. Arrange facilities and amenities.

E. Team Leader and Team Actions (PDCA Implementation Phase)
   1. Provide Lean Sigma overview training and orientation.
   2. Implement improvements using PDCA process.
   3. Develop follow-up action plans.
   4. Report out as required.

F. Facilitator or Team Leader Actions (Follow-Up Phase)
   1. Follow-up on open action plans.
   2. Complete A3 Project Report and share.
   3. Reward and show appreciation to team members.

G. Management (Follow-Up Phase)
   1. Audit process improvements to goals.

Improve

It is unlikely that 3 or 5 consecutive 8-hour days can be dedicated to the Kaizen Event Part 2 (PDCA Implementation Phase). If this is the case, consider segmenting the activities into 4-hour increments over a 1 - 2 month period. If this is not feasible, consider detailing each improvement initiative as a separate project. Whatever time frame is used for your Kaizen Event, ensure all improvement activities (process changes) follow the PDCA process.

The following benefits can be obtained by conducting a Kaizen Event:

> ❖ Meet improvement needs that are urgent or at crisis level
> ❖ Allow for focused improvements in a specific period of time due to that area being in continual use
> ❖ Achieve significant changes in minimal time

Note: Depending on the team's availability prior to Part 2. PDCA Implementation Phase, some activities (i.e., creating a process or value stream map, collecting cycle times, conducting the Waste Walk, etc.) can be done prior to this phase.

Sensei Tips for Kaizen Events

> ❖ The Planning Phase is paramount for a successful Kaizen Event of any type.
> ❖ Communicate to process area employees that are not on the improvement team.

❖ Do not surprise management with major issues or changes during any part of the Kaizen Event.

❖ Be flexible about the type of Kaizen Event. The various team types are:

Standard 5 (or 3 Day) Kaizen - The PDCA Implementation Phase allocates 3 to 5 days for the beta or pilot of process changes.

Rolling Kaizen - All meetings and process changes spread over 3 months.

Today's Kaizen - All phase meetings are within a 4 week timeframe as well as solutions to the known problem or continuous improvement initiative are implemented.

Web Based Kaizen - All meetings are conducted via Web conferencing communication applications (Huddle, Skype, Infinite Conferencing, GoToMeeting, etc.).

❖ Each type of Kaizen Event is comprised of similar activities. However, each type may have a slightly different approach. Become familiar with all types and determine the one that provides the most value to your organization.

A team created the following Kaizen Event templates for their Standard 5 Day Kaizen Event:

Kaizen Event Preparation Schedule

The Kaizen Event Preparation Schedule should be used by the Team Leader, Black Belt, or whomever is facilitating the continuous improvement event. The success of a Kaizen Event depends on the detailed planning that is done beforehand. Place a checkmark (✔) by those items that have been completed.

3 Weeks Before Event

❏ 1. Select area and topic.
❏ 2. Meet with Sponsor (Champion), Process Owner, Financial Leader, and any other key associates to
   - Prioritize value streams that relate to Balanced Scorecard or Performance Dashboard
   - Secure full time participation by team members for the event
   - Ensure Sponsor is available for the kick-off meeting and the report outs (if applicable)
   - Discuss objectives and scope of the project
❏ 3. Ask these questions:
   - Will this team improve the process/functional performance?
   - Are the resources being focused on the right priorities?
   - What is the business case for analyzing and improving this value stream?
❏ 4. When filling out a Team Charter, ensure:
   - Facilitator is assigned
   - Additional expertise (i.e., Black Belt, Lean Sensei, etc.) is available (if necessary)
   - Team member roles are defined (scribe, timekeeper, etc.)
   - Boundaries of the project are clearly defined
   - Customers of the process are clearly identified
   - Suppliers to the process or area are clearly identified
   - Dates have been established and agreed to
❏ 5. Secure conference room for the event. The room should be:
   - Located as close as possible to the process area that is being worked on
   - Available for the duration of the event
   - Large enough to conduct simulations (if required in the training)
❏ 6. Obtain all necessary supplies, such as:
   - Post-it Notes
   - Posts-it Self-Stick Easel Pad
   - Catering requirements
   - Flip charts and markers
   - Access to copy machine
   - Materials (pocket guides)
   - LCD projector
   - Copies of training
   - Snacks ☺

Deliverables

❏ 1. Team Charter created.
❏ 2. Metric/goal initially agreed upon.
❏ 3. Date(s) of the event determined.
❏ 4. Invitation sent to team members that includes date, location, event particulars, and Team Charter.
❏ 5. All necessary supplies (training materials) have been ordered.

Comments/Notes:

_____

_____

Improve

This Kaizen Event Preparation Schedule for the Planning Phase allows for good project management techniques.

Kaizen Event Preparation Schedule

The Kaizen Event Preparation Schedule should be used by the Team Leader, Black Belt, or whomever is facilitating the continuous improvement event. The success of a Kaizen Event depends on the detailed planning that is done beforehand. Place a checkmark (✔) by those items that have been completed.

2 Weeks Before Event

☐ 1. Review the 3 Weeks Before Event list.
☐ 2. Gather data/identify sources that would be on a current state value stream or process map.
- Obtain financials, flowcharts, etc. of the process(es)
- Run reports of data of the current process or collect real-time data (if applicable)
☐ 3. Determine current customer steady state demand (takt time).
☐ 4. Determine key individuals needed to support the event as on an ad hoc basis (facilities, IT, etc.). Communicate with them appropriately.
☐ 5. Review the Team Charter with sponsor and process owner. Discuss schedules, measurements, targets, and deliverables on the proposed event.
☐ 6. Review Lessons Learned, Sunset Reports, and Kaizen Event Evaluation Forms from any previous events that may impact this event.

Deliverables

☐ 1. Team Charter completed and agreement reached on specific deliverables.
☐ 2. Sponsor scheduled for kick-off meeting and report outs.
☐ 3. Date(s) of the event determined.
☐ 4. All team members notified.
☐ 5. Data collection started.

1 Week Before Event

☐ 1. Review 3 Weeks Before Event and 2 Weeks Before Event list and resolve open issues.
☐ 2. Hold final preparation meeting with process owner.
☐ 3. Review metrics and goals with process owner for final agreement.
☐ 4. Update Team Charter, if necessary.

Deliverables

☐ 1. Team member participation verified.
☐ 2. Team Charter released to all team members.
☐ 3. Materials acquired.
☐ 4. Room and catering verified (those snacks ☺).

Comments/Notes:

_____

_____

This Kaizen Event Preparation Schedule for the Planning Phase allows for good project management techniques to be continued.

Kaizen Event Scorecard

The Kaizen Event Scorecard conveys improvement results. It provides the team with necessary data to make corrections on negative trends if improvements are not going as expected. The Scorecard provides management with progress-to-date.

Event Name: Site/Location: Date:

Value Stream Impacted: Process Owner(s):   Team Members:

Team Champion/Sponsor: Team Leader:

Measurements	Metrics							
	# Start of Event	# End of Event	7 Day Date: ___	14 Day Date: ___	30 Day Date: ___	60 Day Date: ___	90 Day Date: ___	Target

Overall Evaluation:

R Y G	R Y G	R Y G	R Y G	R Y G

Key: ■ Performance Meets or Exceeds Target (Green)
       Performance is Short but close to Target (within 10% of Target) (Yellow)
       Performance is Significantly Unfavorable to Target (below 10% of Target) (Red)

If a measurement is not meeting the target, use the below 4 W's (What, Who, When, and Why) to clearly indicate how you plan to meet or exceed target.

What	Who	When	Why

Comments/Notes:

This Kaizen Event Scorecard for the Follow-Up Phase assists the team to focus on the 7, 14, 30+ days measurements. This is critical to ensure the improvements are sustained - as metrics drive behavior.

Note: These three forms are from a subset of over 30+ worksheets from the books *Kaizen Demystified* and *Kaizen Demystified for Healthcare* and are available at TheLeanStore.com under Etools for the industry segment.

Improve

Plan-Do-Check-Act (PDCA) Process

Good, Better Best,
Never let them rest,
Til the Good becomes Better and
Better becomes Best!

Anonymous

What is it?

PDCA is an interactive four-step problem solving and improvement process, typically used to implement business process improvements. PDCA or Plan-Do-Check-Act is also known as the Deming or Shewhart cycle. Numerous mini-improvements may need to be implemented to meet the deliverables as defined in the Team Charter. Subsequently, mini-improvements should be defined using the tools of VA versus NVA Analysis, Histograms, 5 Why Analysis, Force Field Analysis, Impact Maps, etc. For these improvements to be implemented and verified as to their effectiveness, the use of the PDCA process may be used. The PDCA is complimentary to the D-M-A-I-C and other problem solving and continuous improvement methodologies.

What is it?

PDCAs are sometimes referred to as experiments or trials. The process and terms help people commit or "buy-in" to trying something new. Getting people to try something new is one of the more challenging parts of reaching an improved (or future) state. Use of a PDCA experiment or trial is a short-term, controlled trial process, used to capture data and learn about the process. This approach helps people adapt to change more easily. Once the PDCA improvement has been proven successful, the necessary standards need to be updated or created.

℞ How do you do it?

The following steps or guidelines define the PDCA process:

1. Plan – Define the improvement action plan or experiment. What will be done, who will do it, and how will it be measured? Document this information.

2. Do – Implement the improvement plan or experiment.

3. Check – Check that the intended improvement was realized. Measure and discuss the results of the experiment with the team and process workers involved.

4. Act – Act to standardize the new process if the improvement improved performance. Act to put the process back to its original condition if the experiment did not improve performance. Determine how and why it did not work and begin at (1) Plan again.

Use the Action Item Log previously described to document and track the progress of PDCA activities. Continuous and incremental improvements will be realized as each successive PDCA is completed.

The following benefits can be obtained by following the PDCA process:

❖ Minimize possibility of error
❖ Allow for real-time corrective action
❖ Optimize the utilization of time
❖ Improve productivity immediately

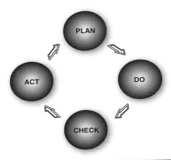

Improve

Sensei Tips for PDCA

Teams must work to ensure good communication occurs prior to and during all PDCA improvements.

Action Plan

Action Item List - Kaizen Event Phlebotomy

Effective Sept 21

Event	Project	Do-It	#	Description	Who	Plan Priority	Plan Date	Comments	Date Complete
			1	Recollect Cell (Immediate notification of recollect to office)	C. Barber	LH	Oct	Reduce QNS draws + manual loads. Improve result quality + increase satisfaction. Ensure that all communication re: recollects occurs within 24 hrs.	
			2	Phlebotomy Standard Work-Central Draw	Phleb. Mgr	HL	Nov	Quicker TAT, more accurate specimens, standardize technique	
			3	Processing/Load Automation standard work	RRC Mgr	HL	Nov	Triage answer tube, sort to appropriate racks + load automation	
			4	Hematology Flow Cell	Hemo Mgr	HL	Sept	Improve productivity at one station, thereby avoiding extra walking and errors	
			5	Courier standard work	Matt	HL	Sept	Couriers make more pickups from offices therefore making more drop-offs to lab. Quicker TAT	
			6	Lab Works – Increase Rollout	Lab Mgr	HL	Oct	This will save time by less double labelling. Drs. office will have labels directly sent to them	
			7	Frequency of Packaging	Office Mgr	HL	Nov	Allows courier to pick up more often (2X), Quicker results	
			8	Immunology - Shared Specimens	Dr. Aslakson	HL	Sept	Insure that all testing gets done in a timely manner without the need to hunt & search for testing	
			9	Manual Hemotology	RRL Mgr	LL	Sept	Consistent processing of batched manual tests. i.e., ESR every 2 hours. Storage rack systems (check completeness)	
			10	Relabel Manual Chem	RRL Mgr	LL	Oct	Samples should be labeled for HgbAcc prior to sending to Chemistry Analyzer	

This Kaizen Event Phlebotomy team separated their improvement project into three parts (note the left three columns): (1) activities to be done during the formal Kaizen "Event" time, (2) activities that warrant a separate "Project," and (3) activities to be done prior to the Event, (Just) "Do It."

5S

If you can't do 5S, forget all the rest!
Anonymous

What is it?

5S *ensures physical areas and paper-based or electronic documents are systematically kept clean and organized.* This assures employee safety in meeting customer expectations while providing the foundation to build a Lean Sigma organization. The five steps for 5S are:

Step 1 - Sort
Step 2 - Set-In-Order
Step 3 - Shine (or Scrub)
Step 4 - Standardize
Step 5 - Sustain

The systematic 5-step process makes 5S unique and successful in many different industries.

What does it do?

5S provides an opportunity to involve all employees in the Lean Sigma process. 5S is a simple and common-sense approach to improving a process or work area.

In today's business environment, as well as in every industry, there are three inter-related business areas: (1) physical elements such as work cubicles, doors, aisle ways, equipment, supplies, etc., (2) paper-based elements such as forms, work documents, labs, orders, prescriptons, etc. and (3) electronic documents such as emails, , EMR reports, text messages, spreadsheets, hyperlinks to information, bookmarks, and smart phone and tablet communications, etc. The basic principles of 5S equally apply to all three.

Improve

How do you do it?

The following steps or guidelines are used when implementing 5S:

Step 1 - Sort

Sort *weeds out items that have not been used for a period of time or are not expected to be used.* The team and/or worker should follow these steps:

a. Select an area or process to apply the 5S tool if not defined as an improvement activity within the Project or Team Charter. Ensure that the process or area is large enough to make a difference, but small enough to complete with the resources available.

b. Agree on the purpose of the area or process being considered. Agree on what belongs and what does not belong in the area. Consider creating a Red Tag staging area to remove items that do not belong. Create a group-wide Red Tag folder for any electronic documents that needed to be removed from email folders, C: drives, etc. before file standards are created. It may be necessary to train employees on effective use of Windows Explorer or functionality with the EMR System. The Red Tag area or folder can be used to determine further disposition of items.

c. Take before photos of the area or screen shots of the files/folders.

d. Remove all physical items or electronic documents from the area or folder as determined in (b). A color-coding system is used for an item or file: needed - but needs to move (green), not needed (red), and not sure - need additional input or approval (yellow).

e. Determine disposition of all items.

Note: Many software applications assign color-codes to track frequency and use of electronic files.

Step 2 - Set-In-Order
Set-In-Order *establishes locations where items belong with labels or visual markings.* The team and/or worker should follow these steps:

a. Create the appropriate visual indicators to label and identify all items in the area. This will ensure that items or files removed from the area can "find" its way back. Electronic files include bookmarks, hyperlinks, shared-directory file protections, filename conventions, etc.

b. Use visual controls and visual management principles. For example, the following color-coding system may be used for physical items in an organization for both service and administrative areas:

- ❖ Yellow = General caution
- ❖ Red = Urgent items or areas
- ❖ Green = Good or on-target items
- ❖ Orange = Moveable equipment, parking spots
- ❖ Blue = Incoming orders or items
- ❖ Yellow w/ Black Strip = Safety Warnings

Step 3 - Shine (or Scrub)
Shine *cleans the area and establishes a sequence to maintain the area.* This may include cleaning the keyboard and shampooing the floor mats every month, to running a disk utilization program. The team should do "spring cleaning," then create a standard cleaning plan. The team and/or worker should follow these steps:

a. Clean items that will remain in the area. Clean and dust physical spaces; paint, polish, and restore items "like the day they were new!" This applies to offices, public spaces, and equipment. Attention to detail now helps you spot abnormalities and waste.

b. Ask your team why the area cannot be kept in this condition, what it would take to keep it in this condition, why can we never find the right file in our shared directory, why do we have so many versions of the same file, etc. The 5S discipline is the foundation for all continuous improvement projects!

c. Use the information gathered from steps 1 - 3 for the 4th and 5th S.

d. Ensure the area is "cleaned" out on a regular basis. Regularly purging your file system will save you time in retrieving files when they are required. This helps eliminate wastes of motion and file inventory.

Improve

Step 4 - Standardize
Standardize creates guidelines or protocols to keep an area organized, orderly, and clean (or scrubbed). Make standards visual and obvious. The team and/or worker should follow these steps:

a. List specific tasks and locations from the Set-In-Order and Shine steps.

b. List who will perform tasks.

c. List required frequency and resources required.

d. Ensure everyone has access to the task list.

Step 5 - Sustain
Sustain creates an auditing process to ensure a long-term adherence to standards. Nearly all 5S and Lean Sigma projects begins with initial enthusiasm for change; however, today's standards require continuous improvement. The team and/or worker should follow these steps to ensure the 5S system is sustained:

a. Create an audit team. Designated internal auditor(s) will provide an unbiased evaluation on how 5S is working.

b. Create a 5S Audit check sheet. List the specific attributes to be audited from the information derived from the 3rd and 4th S.

c. Identify the frequency of audits. Typically, once a month is sufficient for the independent audit team and once per week for any individual self-assessment.

d. Follow the five-level Likert item scale for audit responses to each question or statement:

1 - Strongly Disagree (or unacceptable, needs immediate improvement)
2 - Disagree (or needs improvement)
3 - Neither Agree nor Disagree (or OK, meets minimum requirements)
4 - Agree (or meets and sometimes exceeds requiremens)
5 - Strongly Agree (or constantly exceeds requirements and use as an example of excellence)

Provide a Scoring Legend once an audit is complete. A suggested Scoring Legend follows: (E.g., you may have 20 audit-type questions or statements, each with a value of 5 points each, or 25 questions, each with a value of 4 points each, etc.)

80 - 100   Doing Well - Keep up the good work
60 - 79   Doing OK - Must make more effort
<60   Not So Good - Very little effort shown

Whatever your scoring system, remember to be as positive and supportive as possible. Low scores may indicate that the person (or group) requires more information, support, and/or training.

e. Communicate overall success to the group. Praise those that adhere to the process. Communicate privately to those that do not adhere to the process and address their concerns.

The following benefits can be obtained by implementing 5S:

- ❖ Minimize waste throughout the process or area
- ❖ Allow for an understanding of the importance of standards
- ❖ Ensure employee participation and involvement
- ❖ Improve productivity immediately
- ❖ Help to ensure good quality and work consistency

Improve

Sensei Tips for 5S

The following photos are various stages of 5S:

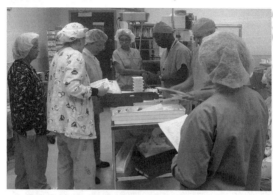

(Sort) Create Sorting Guidelines (forward person holding such guidelines) so team members are aware of what stays and what does not.

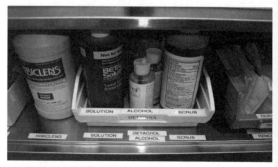

(Set-In-Order) Ensure labels are also placed on the removable containers where the supply resides.

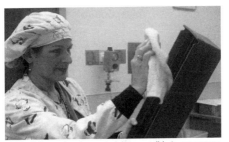

(Shine) Keep cleaning materials accessible to encourage cleanliness.

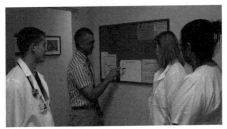

(Standardize) Post 5S standards. Alert all staff to expectations.

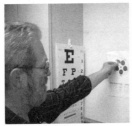

(Sustain) Audits and recognition will help keep the 5S program alive.

Improve

Visual Controls

*Build up your weaknesses until they become
your strong points.*
Knute Rockne

What is it?

Visual control is a technique employed whereby control of an activity or process is made easier or more effective by deliberate use of visual signals (signs, information displays, maps, layouts, instructions, alarms, and poka-yoke or mistake proofing devices). These signals can be of many forms, from simple signs in a lobby area and different function keys on the keyboard, to various types of measurements about a problem or departmental goal, to kanbans and heijunka boxes; these signals can also be audio. A visual control effectively communicates the information needed for decision-making.

What does it do?

Visual controls are part of an overall communication system (a picture is worth a thousand words) of an organization. Visual controls will ensure standards are met and work is completed on time to continue to the next process without errors. Visual controls should be used (or at least considered) at every juncture of the Lean Sigma project. Visual controls are used to identify conditions that may cause an error, or if an error occurs, what must be done to prevent it from becoming a defect.

The four levels of visual controls are as follows:

Level 1 - Indicators: provide information about the immediate environment, area, department, or process. These indicators are passive and people may or may not notice them or respond to them. It is the simplest form to influence or change behavior. Examples of Level 1 visual controls are:

- ❖ "Allergy Alert" is highlighted in red on the patient's chart and ID bracelet
- ❖ Signs, posters, maps, arrows, lines on floors,etc.
- ❖ Color-coding emails or other electronic files and folders
- ❖ Rainbow draws

Level 2 - Signals: *cause a visual or auditory alarm that grabs your attention and warns that a mistake or error may occur.* Signals have a higher level of influencing behavior. People may ignore these, but are aware that something may be wrong. Examples of Level 2 visual controls are:

- ❖ Andon lights
- ❖ Audible "beep" when bar code scans properly
- ❖ An "alert" would occur signaling a possible drug interaction as a patient's medications are typed
- ❖ Performance Dashboards on Desktop screens
- ❖ "Radiation in Use" alarms (flashing red light)
- ❖ A sound (or chirp) from the copy machine indicating service is required or ink is low

Level 3 - Controls: *physical or electronic limit prevents something from occurring due to the negative impact it will have on the process (or area).* These are more aggressive than Levels 1 and 2, and guide and control behaviors so that only the correct option is selected. Examples of Level 3 visual controls are:

- ❖ Fingerprint swipe on PYXIS machine
- ❖ Pre-surgical checklists and "time-out" in OR
- ❖ Locks, security codes, RFIDs, etc.
- ❖ Email rules and filters
- ❖ Drop-down menu selections
- ❖ Heparin packaging - adult versus pediatric doses
- ❖ Child-proof medicine caps
- ❖ Ready to fill safety syringes

Level 4 - Guarantees: *ensure that correct decisions are made.* They are the highest level of visual control (most likely referred to as mistake proofing devices). Visual guarantees force the correct decisions to be made. Examples of Level 4 visual controls are:

- ❖ Mechanical wall connections for gases, such as oxygen and nitrogen
- ❖ Swipe cards for secure entry or time keeping
- ❖ Usernames and passwords to an account
- ❖ Safety cutters for orthopedics

Improve

When creating a signaling device, a physical or electronic visual control, decide which level is most appropriate for the situation. Clearly, Levels 3 and 4 are the most comprehensive in terms of ensuring that an error or mistake does not occur. The solution may not always be possible or cost effective. Consider information requirements and availability both upstream and downstream of the area being addressed. Once the process requirement has been determined, select the most effective level of visual control. Implement visual controls in a PDCA fashion to ensure success.

The following chart summarizes the visual control levels and examples:

Attribute	Type of Device			
	Level 1 - Indicators	Level 2 - Signals	Level 3 - Controls	Level 4 - Guarantees
Power Level	Lowest Passive Only tells	Low-Medium Assertive Grabs senses	Medium-High Aggressive Narrows options	High Assured Allows only the correct response
Impact on Behavior	Influences Informs Indicates Shows Suggests	Alerts Alarms Warns Signals Prompts Announces	Directs Guides Limits Guards Restricts Restrains Hinders	Compels Forces Ensures Prohibits Inhibits Eliminates Guarantees
Road Examples	Road signs	Road lights	Road barriers	Road designs
Workplace Examples	Signs Posters Pictures Lists Maps Arrows Color-coding Bar Charts	Alarms Buzzers Horns Music Lights Counters Bells Performance Dashboards	One-way turn styles Container size File space Guarding Ropes Drop-down menus	Locks Automatic operations Rules/filters Username/passwords

R_x *How do you do it?*

The following steps or guidelines are used to create a visual control:

1. Select an area or process to apply visual controls.
Lean Six Sigma projects require visual controls. Creating and maintaining visual controls can be challenging and fun at the same time.

2. Identify the process requirements and information that needs to be shared.
If the process is used by other co-workers, ensure they have input into creating the visual control. Ask critical questions: "What information is needed?" and "What information needs to be shared for the process to run properly?"

3. Develop visual controls.
Develop visual controls that provide the information needed and information to be shared in such a way as to make the information available at-a-glance. Provide training for upstream, downstream, and area workers regarding the meaning of the visual controls. Make sure everyone understands the visual controls and uses them as intended.

4. Implement the visual controls using the PDCA process.
Visual controls may require beta testing or experimentation to ensure they meet process requirements. Ensure a logical implementation methodology is used, such as the PDCA. As part of the PDCA implementation process, it is recommended that after any new visual control is implemented that the improvement team provides the appropriate follow-up and checks the effectiveness of the improvement. If the improvement is working, work to standardize the process. If the improvement requires adjustment, take the necessary action, and continue to monitor the improvement.

The following benefits can be obtained by using visual controls:

- ❖ Reduce confusion in completing a process
- ❖ Reduce opportunity for errors and defects (using mistake proofing) to improve quality
- ❖ Assist in adhering to a process standard
- ❖ Improve efficiency and customer satisfaction

Improve

Sensei Tips for Visual Controls

The following are examples of visual controls:

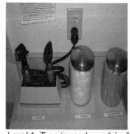

Level 1 -Tape is used as a "sign" to "inform" staff where items are to be returned.

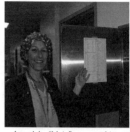

Level 1 - "Lists" are used to "indicate" what items belong at a location.

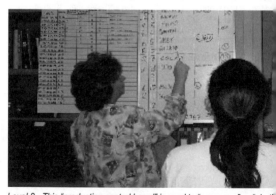

Level 2 - This "production control board" is used to "announce" or "alert" the nursing supervisor if additional staff is needed to meet patient flow requirements. A visual control does not have to be fancy or high-tech!

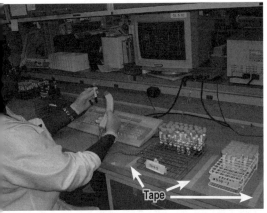

Level 3 - Tape is used to denote the "container size" that "limits" the work in the queue.

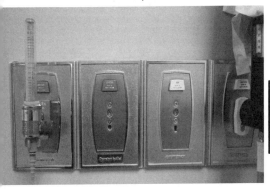

Level 4 - Different valve connectors "ensure" that the oxygen and nitrogen hoses are connected to the right valve ports. For example, a nitrogen hose cannot be connected to the oxygen wall connector valve and vice versa.

Improve

Mistake Proofing

When you're out of quality,
you're out of business.

Unknown

What is it?

Mistake proofing is a system designed to ensure that it i.
impossible to make a mistake or produce a defect. Mistake
proofing is also known as error proofing. The Japanese term, poka
yoke, is derived from "poka" - inadvertent mistake and "yoke" - avoid. /
poka-yoke device is any physical or electronic mechanism that prevent
a mistake from being made or ensures that if a mistake is made it i
obvious at a glance. Poka-yoke ensures subsequent actions from
becoming defects. Defects are caused by process errors, equipmer
and material errors, and worker errors; defects are the results of those
errors. Mistakes will not turn into defects if they are discovered and
eliminated beforehand. Defects occur because of errors; the two have a
cause-and-effect relationship. However, errors will not turn into defects
feedback and action takes place prior to the error stage. Visual controls
(previous section) play a large role in reducing the opportunity for error
occurrence, thereby ensuring that no defects result from the process.

Defects vs. Errors

To be a defect:

- The process or service deviates from specifications or standards of service.

- The process or service does not meet customer (internal or external) expectations.

To be an error:

- An action in the process deviates from an intended action, or an action is not performed or another action is performed instead of the required one.

- All defects are created by errors, but not all errors result in defects.

What does it do?

Mistakes or errors are waste. Mistakes or errors not only cause a process to be repeated and corrected, assume they create customer ill will. Generally, a typical dissatisfied customer will tell eight to ten people about a problem. One in five will tell twenty. It takes twelve positive incidents to make up for one negative incident.

Apply mistake proofing methods: (1) before the process starts, (2) during the process itself, and (3) immediately after the process has been completed.

Elimination of errors through mistake proofing is the foundation of Lean Sigma methods. Mistake proofing techniques and devices help avoid costly errors and customer disappointments. Mistake proofing devices limit errors and help to encourage the correct behavior of a process. Reasons for errors follow:

1. Requests of inappropriate or unknown procedures, processes, or standards
2. Variability in the operations and processes
3. Wrong, inaccurate, damaged, or excessively variable inputs
4. Lack of proper communication of requirements and expectations
5. Human error – forgetting to do part of the process, doing part of the process incorrectly, or using the incorrect information or data to complete a process

Human error is the most difficult defect to eliminate and occurs for a variety of reasons. Human errors occur because we are not machines. They are difficult to avoid. The key to mistake proofing is to develop processes in which errors can be prevented, detected, and/or corrected before they are passed on to downstream activities.

Example follows:

The necessity of training farm hands for first class farms in the fatherly handling of farm livestock is foremost in the eyes of farm owners. Since the forefathers of farm owners trained the farm hands for first class farms in a fatherly handling of farm livestock, the farm owners feel they should carry on with family tradition of training farm hands of first class farmers in the fatherly handling of farm livestock because they believe it is the basis of good fundamental farm management.

Improve

There are 36 "f's" in the paragraph as shown in the following paragraph.

The necessity of training farm hands for first class farms in the fatherly handling of farm livestock is foremost in the eyes of farm owners. Since the forefathers of farm owners trained the farm hands for first class farms in a fatherly handling of farm livestock, the farm owners feel they should carry on with family tradition of training farm hands of first class farmers in the fatherly handling of farm livestock because they believe it is the basis of good fundamental farm management.

If you followed a standard process of counting the "f's" in a row, then the sum for the totals from each row may have been more accurate.

Row 1 = 6
Row 2 = 5
Row 3 = 7
Row 4 = 6
Row 5 = 5
Row 6 = 4
Row 7 = 3

Total = 36

One way of mistake proofing a human process is to establish a formal or standard process (e.g., for counting). Other forms of mistake proofing are redundancy checks where multiple workers will check and re-check or ask for the same information. Examples of mistake proofing are:

- ❖ Surgical patients mark the intended surgery area with a pen to ensure the surgeon works on the correct area once the patient is under anesthesia
- ❖ Double-check administration of insulin
- ❖ Double-check administration of blood and blood products
- ❖ Use a Surgical Safety Checklist to reduce morbidity and mortality

℞ How do you do it?

The following steps or guidelines are used to create mistake proofing devices or systems:

1. Shift your paradigm.
Errors can be prevented! Begin looking for the source of defects, not just the defects themselves. Look for opportunities to eliminate them at their source. The root cause of defects is in the process, not the people.

2. Conduct analysis.
To analyze the problem identify and describe the defect or potential error in-depth, including the rate that it may have been occurred over time. A Failure Prevention Analysis Worksheet (FPAW) can assist in this process. *Failure Prevention Analysis is a technique that allows the team to anticipate potential problems in the solution before implementing any changes, thereby permitting the team to be proactive in preventing any solution(s) from going wrong.* The subsequent processes of mistake proofing will be procedures, visual controls, alarm notifications, etc. that prevent a mistake or to ensure the mistake, if made, is obvious at-a-glance.

The following guidelines help you to create and use the FPAW (see Sensei Tips for an example of this worksheet):

a. Create a list of potential failures for each improvement activity. List the probable cause-effect relationship with any opportunity for error.

b. Rank the potential failures by rating the potential and consequence of each possibility, for each item going wrong. Use a scale from 1 to 5.

c. Multiply the potential and consequence together for each of the potential failures to give the overall rating.

d. Rank each potential failure from highest to lowest (1 - XX).

e. Brainstorm with the team to modify any/all activities to lessen the likelihood of causing a problem.

Improve

Mistake Proofing

3. Standardize the work.

Create or update standard work instructions and train employees to the standards. The standard may already be written (i.e., policy manuals, service standards, work instructions, etc.). Consider offering manuals, instructions, training in pdf or tutorial format on demand for employees

4. Create appropriate visual controls and/or mistake proofing devices or systems.

It may not always be possible to prevent mistakes from happening. Even computer systems can be over-ridden and bar codes ignored. However, the goal must be to reduce the number of defects that are likely to occur. When providing a service (or a unit of work, or a product), ensure the process allows for "making it easy to do the right thing and hard or impossible to do the wrong thing."

The following benefits can be obtained by using mistake proofing devices:

- ❖ Reduce the possibility for errors
- ❖ Make work easier to perform
- ❖ Improve quality
- ❖ Assist adherence to a process standard
- ❖ Improve efficiency
- ❖ Minimize errors and/or reduces their impact

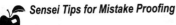

Sensei Tips for Mistake Proofing

The following are examples of mistake proofing:

Failure Prevention Analysis Worksheet

Directions:
1. List all potential failures.
2. Assign a number from 1 to 5 for the potential and consequence of an activity going wrong.
3. Multiply the potential and consequence and rank from highest to lowest.

Potential Rating
1 - Very unlikely to occur - once a year
2 - Might occur rarely - once a month
3 - 50/50 chance to occur within five days
4 - Good chance to occur at least once a day
5 - Excellent chance to occur several times a day

Consequence Rating
1 - Very little or no risk to the patient
2 - Some risk to the patient, but easily corrected
3 - Moderate risk to the patient, needing action
4 - Severe risk to the patient, requiring action
5 - Most severe consequence to the patient, possible death, requiring immediate action

Potential Failure	Potential	Consequence	Overall Rating	Ranking
A. Physicians can't reach PCP for consult (after 15 min. from first call)	3	1	3	5
B. Clerk doesn't see dispo in chart, even though Dr. places it there	1	4	4	4
C. Pt belongings missing, even though form used when pt was in ED	2	4	8	3
D. Quick Reg page prints but is not seen; printer is dedicated	3	4	12	2
E. Transporter still busy with other patients when called for by ED	3	5	15	1

Improvement Solutions:
A. The ED physician would continue with patient care (and admit process) without waiting for PCP call back. ED physician would discuss patient care if and when PCP called back.
B. The team asked the computer support group to investigate whether they could "broadcast" a message to all registrars computer terminals that an ED Admit had been ordered, to assure that the registrars would know that an admit order needed to be processed.
C. The team discussed the possibility that the patient might have additional items of value, besides clothing, that were not noted at the time the form was started; for example, a necklace that was not removed initially, but was then removed for an X-ray. The team decided that training was needed for all staff that came in contact with the patient and the belongings form needed to travel with the patient rather than being placed in the chart.
D. A separate printer had been placed in the Registration area to handle admitting requests from the ED. However, there was still a possibility that a busy registrar might not see the forms immediately, and the audible signal (B) might not be heard in a busy environment.
E. The team added to the unit reporting form a checkbox for transporter being called to remind the Nurse to do that right away. Earlier notification would help the transporter prioritize the work. The team had also piloted the use of a dedicated elevator, which did not seem to be a significant factor at this time, so they discontinued that trial.

Improve

This Failure Prevention Analysis Worksheet details the Potential Failures and addresses each with specific Improvement Solutions.

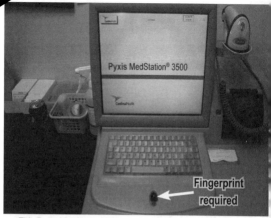

This Pyxis MedStation allows only authorized staff to access the system. Fingerprint identification "prevents" unauthorized users to dispense medication.

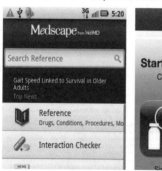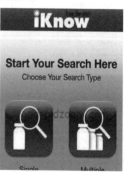

Computer Drug Interaction Checker Software (example of apps shown) that checks for drug interactions is widely available. No harm results if an error is caught by the pharmacist (or system) before the patient receives the medication.

Standard Work

Where there is no standard there can be no Kaizen.
Taiichi Ohno

What is it?

Standard work establishes and controls the best method to complete a task without variation from original intent. Tasks are then executed consistently, without variation, ideally to an established takt time or performance goal. Standard work provides consistent levels of productivity, quality, and safety, and promotes a positive work attitude based on well-documented standards. Standard work, done properly, reduces process variation. It is the basis for all continuous improvement activities.

What does it do?

Standard work is meant to facilitate creativity and innovation by providing a starting point and process for implementing improvements. Standard work improves stability and reduces variation, which are key concepts in Lean Sigma improvement initiatives. The following diagram illustrates the importance of standard work:

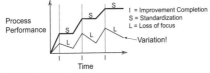

Process Performance / Time

I = Improvement Completion
S = Standardization
L = Loss of focus
Variation!

How do you do it?

The following steps or guidelines are used to create standard work:

1. Define the process. Look for logical beginning and ending points, or repetitive tasks. Make sure to involve the people who do the tasks.

2. Collect timely process data. Gather data from the EMR system using an appropriate sample size. Establish desired task lengths. Best practices may be national benchmarks.

Improve

3. Populate a Time Observation Sheet (commonly referred to as a Cycle Time Worksheet). *A **Time Observation Sheet** is the detailed listing of each activity comprised within the process along with its start and stop times.*

4. Document time observations on a Standard Work Chart. Once the Standard Work Chart has been completed, begin to review the work steps for waste and modify work routing to reduce or eliminate waste. The Standard Work Combination Table may also be used to review process steps influencing takt time, travel time, or processing time. Use a Bar Chart with symbols to represent each process step.

The following benefits can be obtained by creating Standard Work:

- ❖ Eliminate process variation
- ❖ Improve quality
- ❖ Help to ensure takt time (or goal) is met
- ❖ Improve efficiency

Sensei Tips for Standard Work

The following are examples of standard work:

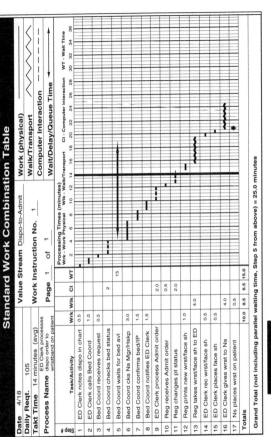

Standard Work Combination Table

Date	4/18			Value Stream	Dispo-to-Admit
Daily Reqt.	105			Work Instruction No.	1
Takt Time	14 minutes (avg)				
Process Name	ED Clerk processes dispo order to wristband on patient			Page	1 of 1

# day	Task/Activity	Wrk	Wlk	CI	WT
1	ED Clerk notes dispo in chart	0.5			
2	ED Clerk calls Bed Coord	1.0			
3	Bed Coord receives request	0.5			
4	Bed Coord checks bed status			2	
5	Bed Coord waits for bed avl				15
6	Bed Coord cks Ns Mgr/Hskp	3.0			
7	Bed Coord confirms bed/IP	1.5			
8	Bed Coord notifies ED Clerk	1.5			
9	ED Clerk process Admit order			2.0	
10	Reg receives Admit order			0.5	
11	Reg changes pt status			2.0	
12	Reg prints new wrst/face sh	1.0			
13	Reg takes wrst/face sh to ED	4.0			
14	ED Clerk rec wrst/face sh	0.5			
15	ED Clerk places face sh	0.5			
16	ED Clerk gives wrst to Ns		4.0		
17	Ns places wrst on patient	0.5			
	Totals	10.0	8.5	6.5	15.0

Grand Total (not including parallel waiting time, Step 5 from above) = 25.0 minutes

Processing Times (minutes)

Wrk – Work Physical   Wlk – Walk/Transport   CI – Computer Interaction   WT – Wait Time

Work (physical) ————
Walk/Transport ∿∿∿∿
Computer Interaction – – –
Wait/Delay/Queue Time ←——→

Improve

This Standard Work Combination Table was for only the wristband process used to get a patient admitted from the ED to an inpatient bed. Subsequent analysis and PDCA would reduce this overall cycle time.

Standard Work Chart

Bed Request		ED Admit to Inpatient Bed Arrival
Process Name		**Value Stream**
ED		ED Staff Lounge (review only)
Department		**Posted Location**

Takt/Pitch	Upstream Process Name	Downstream Process Name
14 minutes	Dispo Written	Admit Order Written

Standard Work Sequence for: Clerk / Bed Control / Reg	Pitch Increment: N/A (Takt Time Used)

1. Clerk receives Dispo order

2. Clerk calls Bed Control

3. Bed Control finds bed

4. Bed Control calls Registration

5. Bed Control calls ED clerk

6. ED Clerk notes bed assignment on Dispo form

7. Registration enters admission in EMR, prints face sheet and wristband

8. Registration brings face sheet and wristband to ED clerk

9. ED clerk places face sheet in chart and gives wristband to Nurse

10. Nurse places wristband on patient

11. Patient is transported to unit

This ED Improvement Team listed all the activities that need to be done on a Standard Work Chart after the Disposition order had been written. They posted the chart in the staff lounge and asked for comments to be written on the chart for one week.

Improving the ED Patient Experience

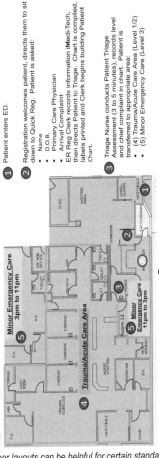

Memorial Healthcare

1. Patient enters ED.

2. Registration welcomes patient, directs them to sit down to Quick Reg. Patient is asked:
   - Name
   - D.O.B.
   - Primary Care Physician
   - Arrival Complaint

   ER Reg Clerk records information (Medi-Tech, then directs Patient to Triage. Chart is compiled, labels printed and Clerk begins building Patient Chart.

3. Triage Nurse conducts Patient Triage Assessment (3 to 5 minutes), records level and chief complaint in chart. Patient is transferred to appropriate area:
   - (4) Trauma/Acute Care Area (Level 1/2)
   - (5) Minor Emergency Care (Level 3)

Minor Emergency Care 3pm to 11pm

Trauma/Acute Care Area

Minor Emergency Care 11pm to 3pm

4 Trauma/Acute Care

Triage Nurse transfers Patient to room and preps for care, e.g., gown, in bed, monitor, then communicates ER process to patient.

Triage Nurse communicates hand off to ER Nurse who completes Bedside Assessment.

Reg Clerk completes full registration.

Treatment and Discharge/Admission

5 Minor Emergency Care

Triage Nurse transfer Patient to room and preps for care, e.g., in bed, elevate a limb, then communicates MEC process to patient.

Triage Nurse communicates hand off to MEC Team who completes Bedside Assessment.

Reg Clerk completes full registration.

MEC Team begins treatment and Discharges Patient

Improve

Floor layouts can be helpful for certain standard work procedures.

Process or Work Area Layout

*If you can't describe what you are doing as a process,
you don't know what you're doing.*
Edward Deming

What is it?

Process or Work Area Layout is the process of reducing the distance between or relocation of resources or people to ensure the product or service is delivered to the customer with minimal or no waste. The basic concept for optimum process or work area layout/relocation is to minimize the wastes of delay, motion, and transportation (total distance traveled by materials or people to complete a process or operation), and to improve flow. To minimize wastes of delay, motion, and transportation, it is common for work areas and processes to be arranged in U or L-shapes to allow for key process workers and materials to be relocated.

What does it do?

U or L-shaped work areas and process flows allow workers in the area to visually see the flow, and connect directly with the upstream process to improve flow. U or L-shaped flows and relocation also allow workers to communicate more effectively as they will typically be in "eye sight and ear shot" from one another. Straight line work areas are common in many "assembly line" type processes and can be represented by the Layout 1 below. Notice the distance between workers and the input and output locations. In a U or L-shaped work area, both workers and materials flow in a circular direction, and the input and output are in close proximity. This enables people to see progress, make needed adjustments, and communicate clearly any developing issues. A U-shaped work area is represented in Layout 2.

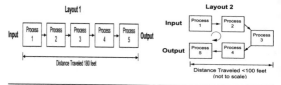

How do you do it?

The following steps or guidelines care used to create or design a new process or work area layout:

1. Review the physical layout and associated process tasks to determine which wastes occur because of the current layout. Consider travel, motion, and delay waste.

2. Brainstorm for reduction or elimination of wastes identified in (1). Processes may need to be modified or standardized and require additional cross-training.

3. Determine the type of flow (i.e., continuous flow, paced flow, or scheduled flow) that will support (2). (See pages 177 - 178.)

4. Determine the flow tool (i.e., Heijunka Leveling, Pull Systems and Kanbans, Supermarkets, or FIFO Lanes) that will support the type of flow. (See pages 179 - 189.)

5. Obtain management approval, commitment, and support.

6. Implement the new layout using the PDCA process at a time that minimizes disruption to the area. Post new standards when new layout is completed. Kaizen Events may work well for this step.

7. Balance workloads among workers and train accordingly.

8. Consider new technologies and software enhancements as you continue to improve.

The following benefits can be obtained by creating or designing a new process or work area layout:

- ❖ Ensure most efficient movement of people, information, and materials
- ❖ Improve communications among processes
- ❖ Improve efficiency of equipment, people, and materials
- ❖ Provide greater job flexibility if someone is absent

Improve

Sensei Tips for Process or Work Area Layout

The following are examples of process or work area layouts:

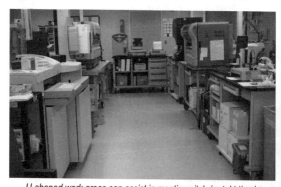

U-shaped work areas can assist in meeting pitch (or takt time). One clinician working multiple instruments situated in a U-shaped configuration saves valuable time and reduces wait time and unnecessary transportation, while expediting critical testing (value-added time). A WIN-WIN scenario for the laboratory, clinician, and patient.

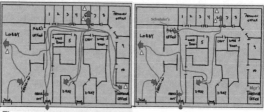

The current state at this Orthopedic's practice (left photo) from patient arrival to next scheduled appointment shows numerous back-and-forths. The average wait time was 67 minutes with a standard deviation of 59 minutes. After Lean flow was implemented, the future state (right photo) shows a large reduction in patient travel. The average wait time in this new Lean state is 29 minutes with a standard deviation of 16 minutes.

Mass Customization

You can have any color as long as it is black.
Henry Ford

What is it?

Mass customization combines the low costs of mass production processes with the variable output required to meet individual customer needs. Some examples of mass customization are fast food restaurants. Fast food restaurants combine a variety of products with standard processes and order combinations to allow their customers to determine choices on the spot with quick and efficient order/service request fulfillment. In healthcare, mass customization is demonstrated by surgical and med carts, certain supply items, as well as certain scheduling systems. EMR, patient care protocols (e.g., AMICHF, stroke, etc.), care transitions, etc. also exhibit mass customization characteristics.

What does it do?

Application of mass customization to healthcare functions improves throughput and turnaround times. Mass customization combines standardization and economies of scale to a process or service.

How do you do it?

The following steps or guidelines are used to determine whether principles of mass customization apply:

1. Create a process flow diagram or value stream map noting process variations/options and volumes, if known.

2. Complete a volume and mix Pareto Chart analysis.

3. Review the process flow diagram or value stream map for common and unique sub processes and requirements. Identify points of commonality and difference.

Improve

4. Develop a plan to stage physical or electronic requirements to a point immediately upstream of differentiation and or develop a plan to deliver all possible options at customer demand.

5. As new demand occurs, pull from staged requirements (build to order), create differentiation, and deliver products or services as required.

The following benefits can be obtained by using the concept of mass customization:

- ❖ Reduce inventories and queue times
- ❖ Allow more options for the customer with greater speed of delivery for product or service
- ❖ Leverage existing organizational and value-chain resources
- ❖ Allow customers to identify or build solutions to their own needs

 Sensei Tips for Mass Customization

The following are examples of mass customization:

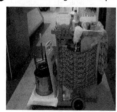 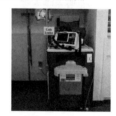

Pre-staging items, supplies, equipment, etc. is a form of mass customization (e.g., Housekeeping and Crash Carts). Also, surgical carts and trays can be a form of mass customization.

New from template
Calendar Wizard
Normal
General Templates...
Templates on my Web Sites...
Templates on Microsoft.com

Templates used in software applications can be a form of mass customization.

Flow

When everything seems to be going against you, remember that the airplane takes off against the wind, not with it.

Henry Ford

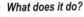

What is it?

There are several ways to improve service and workflow to reduce waste and possibly improve customer satisfaction. This section outlines three flow methods and four flow tools that can be used to create a smooth workflow. It is important to note that in reality, many flows are a combination of these methods and tools. The goal of Lean flow is to reduce batch sizes. This will minimize Work-In-Progress (WIP).

What does it do?

Flow Methods

There are three basic flow methods:

1. Continuous (or One-Piece) Flow
2. Paced Flow
3. Scheduled Flow

1. Continuous (or One Piece) Flow

Continuous flow *is when customer orders or demands are initiated and the process continues uninterrupted until the orders or demands are satisfied.* Examples of continuous flow processes in healthcare are Level I trauma, stat lab orders, surgical procedures, labor and delivery, etc.

Continuous flow is most successful when the following conditions exist:

❖ Order Urgency = High
❖ Order Pattern = Irregular or unpredictable
❖ Order Fulfillment Process = Predictable or standardized

Improve

2. Paced Flow

Paced flow *processing is used where customer order fulfillment tasks are done with regular frequency on a timed schedule.* Examples of paced flow processes in healthcare are physician rounds at specified times throughout the day, dispensing medications, lab pick-ups, dietary delivery and pick-ups. In these cases, items, patients, or required services at specific times are cycled. Paced flow can be leveled by volume or process type.

Paced flow is most successful when the following conditions exist:

- ❖ Order Urgency = Medium
- ❖ Order Pattern = Regular and predictable
- ❖ Order Fulfillment Process = Predicable or standardized

3. Scheduled Flow

Scheduled flow *is where customer orders or demands are known or predicted and then scheduled or reserved for fulfillment at a specific time.* Examples of scheduled flow processes in healthcare are surgeries, physician appointments, dialysis treatments, chemotherapy, and MRIs. Clients, customers, or patients call to request an appointment (or product delivery) for a specific time and date. A schedule is maintained by the service provider.

Scheduled flow is most successful when the following conditions exist:

- ❖ Order Urgency = Low
- ❖ Order Pattern = Irregular or unpredictable
- ❖ Order Fulfillment Process = Unpredictable or non-standard

Pitch *is the adjusted takt time that establishes an optimal and smooth workflow throughout the value stream.* Pitch can be used to regulate workflow using any of these three flow methods. In other words, pitch is the adjusted takt time (or multiple of) when takt time is too short. You can also think of this as efficient small-lot batching. (Note: batching 'per se' is non-Lean.)

Examples of pitch in healthcare may include such things as physician rounds, dispersing meds on the floor, meal deliveries, shifting or turning patients to prevent bed sores, call-backs, prescription calls to pharmacy, and spinning of blood tubes.

Flow Tools

The four basic flow tools are:

1. Heijunka Leveling
2. Pull Systems and Kanbans
3. Supermarkets
4. First-In First-Out (FIFO) Lanes

1. Heijunka Leveling

Heijunka Leveling *works to level or smooth flow by delivering goods and/or services in an alternating or patterned manner rather than large chunks of time.* For example, consider the following physician group practice and the three main types of patients to be scheduled:

A = Diabetic patients average 60 minutes due to the complexity of the disease
B = Physicals average 30 minutes (predictable for the most part)
C = Flu visits average 15 minutes (predictable for the most part)

Without Heijunka Leveling:

1 Physician 2 Rooms (w/ Nurse Practitioner or Physician Assistant)
(Scheduling all diabetic patients in am)

	8:00 am	8:30 am	9:00 am	9:30 am	10:00 am	10:30 am	11:00 am	11:30 am	12:30 pm
RM 1	A		A		A		A		
RM 2		A		A		A		A	

	1:00 pm	1:30 pm	2:00 pm	2:30 pm	3:00 pm	3:30 pm	4:00 pm	4:30 pm	5:00 pm
RM 1	B	B	B	B	B	B	B	B	
RM 2	C	C	C	C	C	C	C	C	

The following problems or issues could occur with this type of schedule:

1. If some diabetic patients, due to their acuity, take longer, delays will occur and may impact patient satisfaction. If this occurs near the end of the am schedule, staff may have to work during lunch, thereby increasing costs (i.e., overtime) and staff dissatisfaction.
2. If some diabetic patients finish earlier than expected, there is capacity available (not having shorter visits patients to take up the slack). This will impact productivity.
3. The afternoon pace will be much faster, thereby increasing stress levels for the staff and the possibility for errors.

With Heijunka Leveling:

1 Physician 2 Rooms (w/ Nurse Practitioner or Physician Assistant)
(Scheduling diabetics throughout the day)

	8:00 am	8:30 am	9:00 am	9:30 am	10:00 am	10:30 am	11:00 am	11:30 am	12:30 pm
RM 1	A		A		A		A		
RM 2		B C		B C	B C		B C		

	1:00 pm	1:30 pm	2:00 pm	2:30 pm	3:00 pm	3:30 pm	4:00 pm	4:30 pm	5:00 pm
RM 1	A		A		A		A		
RM 2		B C		B C	B C		B C		

By using Heijunka Leveling the following would most likely occur:

1. Diabetic patients, due to their acuity, take longer, delays are less likely to occur because of shorter patient exam times before the next diabetic patient and the availability of the B/C patients. If this occurs near the end of the am schedule, there should be enough time to ensure everyone finishes at the appropriate time.
2. Diabetic patients that finish earlier than expected, there is capacity available and the B/C patients can be seen. This will have a positive impact on productivity and the bottom-line.
3. The entire day will flow better and stress should be reduced for the staff.

2. Pull Systems and Kanbans

A **Pull System** is a process to ensure nothing is produced upstream (i.e., supplier process) until the downstream (i.e., customer) process "signals" the need for it. This allows the product or service will be provided without detailed schedules. The "signal" for communication in a pull system is referred to as a Kanban, Card, or Kanban Card (or some other type of visual control signal).

Kanbans (pronounced Con – Bons) or "pull signals" are visual (or auditory, electronic, etc.) signals used to control flow and trigger action between processes. Pull signals can be used to identify demand. Bar codes, text messages, service bells or alarms, containers, etc. can be used as a "signal." "Pull signals" help organizations deliver goods and services minimizing waste. The general concept of Kanbans is to regulate work within and between processes, improve flow, minimize stock-outs, and reduce inventories.

Typically, Kanban Cards for supplies contain the following information:

Kanban Re-order Quantity - how much stock needs to be ordered or moved to replenish supplies
Safety Stock Quantity - the reorder point for each Kanban or supply
Restocking Instructions - how the Kanban is placed to ensure correct placement of the Card
Photo of the supply - helps to ensure correct replacement for smaller items and non-common ones
Detailed Item Description - ensures technical aspects of the item are explained
Bar and Item Code - allows for electronic scanning for reordering
Cost per item - allows employees to understand the cost of supplies which can reduce wasteful practices from developing
Ward and Store Locations - the addresses for the storage location

Ensure rules are posted at the location of the Kanban System, if not done electronically.

Examples of Kanban rules are:
1. Move Kanban Cards to order more stock to the Kanban Post. A Kanban Post is the location for the Kanban Cards.
2. Use Kanban Cards to replace the stock.
3. Replace Kanban Cards correctly when restocking.

Other rules may apply to ensure Kanban Card integrity.

Kanbans generally fall into one of the following categories:

1. **Withdrawal Kanban or Move Signal (Card)** indicates that a number of items (i.e., supplies, work-in-process, etc.), electronic files, or documents (orders, labs, etc.) need to be removed or pulled from a location and supplied downstream. A Withdrawal Kanban or Move Signal "pulls" the required items or service from the upstream operation or process and puts them into use.

2. **Supply Kanban or Supply Signal (Card)** indicates the reorder point has been reached due to consumption, and a service, product, supply, electronic document or data needs to be replenished. The Supply Signal authorizes workers to obtain replenishment of what has been consumed from the upstream operation or process.

Improve

3. **Produce Kanban or Delivery Signal (Card)** *indicates that services, supplies, or products need to be produced and/or delivered as a "batch" downstream (typically used by an outside supplier). This can also be referred to as a Signal Kanban.*

The following is an example of a Supply Re-order Kanban:

Item: size 7 latex gloves, 20 used per shift, (3 shifts)
Total usage of size 7 latex gloves for a day: averages 60
Order size: Size 7 latex gloves are purchased in boxes of 100. The additional 40 in a box could be considered a "buffer" for the day. The "buffer" would need to be tracked to ensure no overstocking is done.
Minimum Required: 1 box (100 gloves)
Maximum Required: 3 boxes (300 gloves)
Re-order time from Central Supply: 2 days

Supply Re-order Kanban Card
Item Name: Size #7 latex gloves
Maximum Quantity: 3 boxes - (100 pair/box)
Minimum Quantity: 1 box - (100 pair/box)
Re-order Quantity: 2 boxes   **(Max - Min)**
Vendor Name: Central Supply **Catalog Pg. No:** N/A
Place this card in the Kanban Post

Note: Ensure a Special Order Kanban Card is created and accessible to be filled in by staff for those special order items (e.g., latex free band-aids). Typically there will not be a minimum/maximum number.

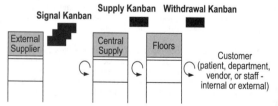

3. Supermarkets

Supermarket describes a specific inventory management process using Kanbans and specified or standard storage locations and package quantities. A Supermarket inventory tool can be used to control flow where make-to-order is not possible. Supermarket is a term taken directly from the inventory management and replenishment system of today's supermarkets. In a modern supermarket, items are provided a specific location, and as items are pulled and purchased by the customers, replenishment is completed to a specified quantity or location. This system ensures that the supermarket rarely runs out of an item and customers never have to wait for replenishment. Supermarkets in healthcare are commonly used for supply items. However, the concept can be used to improve work or patient flow (as shown in the below diagram).

For electronic files and folders a supermarket is a work-controlled method (directory or some other Desktop icon representing work) located between two processes that contain a certain quantity of work or information "buckets" that are "pulled" by the downstream process when needed.

The following is an example of the Supermarket concept being used in the ED. In this scenario, Levels 1 and 2 go directly to an Exam Room. After Quick Reg, patients go to Triage for their assessment. They are assigned an ESI Level of 3, 4, or 5 and proceed to the "Supermarket" or Waiting Room until an Exam Room is available.

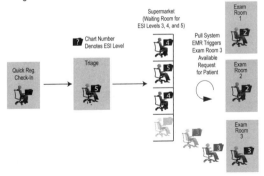

4. First-In First-Out (FIFO)

The **FIFO** system is a work-controlled method which ensure the oldest work (i.e., patient, labs, electronic documents, supply items, etc.) upstream (first-in) is the first to be processed downstream (first-out). For example, nothing frustrates patients more than arriving first, but being assisted last (without due cause and appropriately timed communications).

The team can be creative in establishing the signal method which is typically referred to as a Kanban within the FIFO system to ensure the work is processed as first-in is first-out (or serviced) to the next process. In many patient-related services, this is accomplished by the EMR time stamp when they check-in at the front desk. Ensuring a good FIFO system can be a huge patient satisfier and is known to improve patient satisfaction scores. The important point is to ensure that a signal (Kanban) system is established that works effectively between processes. For example, because lab specimens arrive in groups, a FIFO system will ensure the lab specimens are processed in a timely manner to prevent any specimen spoilage, which would lead to rework (i.e., defect waste). When a FIFO system is full, the upstream process may lend support to the downstream process (if practical) until the work is completed or the service request is met. There is no point in continuing to produce upstream work when the downstream process cannot do anything with it. When this happens, there is overproduction waste, defect waste, etc.

The following is an example of a FIFO system used in most Walk-In (non-emergent) Clinics as well as some Primary Care Offices:

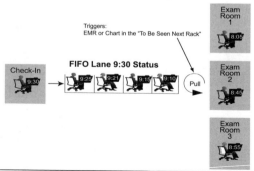

The following is an example of a Kanban System for Surgical Carts:

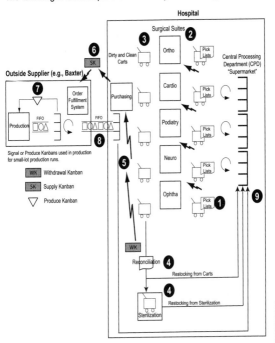

Typically, surgical carts are built 12 to 24 hours before the scheduled surgery. Hospital staff begins prepping for that surgery by pulling the necessary supplies and instruments and placing them in a unique surgical cart for the surgery. Once the Central Processing Department (CPD) gets the surgical confirmation, they print the surgeon's "pick list." This list is like a grocery list and identifies all the supplies and instruments the surgeon will need for the surgery.

Improve

Consider this example on how CPD uses a Kanban approach to supplying and building surgical carts. The following steps are related to the previous diagram on page 185:

1. Once CPD prints the surgical pick list, items are pulled from the surgical kanban and placed on a surgical cart. A Pick List is used to determine which items go on the cart. To minimize and reduce wasted time and supplies, surgeons are encouraged to review and update their "pick lists" on an annual basis (minimally).
2. Completed surgical carts are moved to a holding area near the appropriate OR suite. Pick lists are left with the cart.

3. During surgery, the surgeons focus on the task at hand, techs place used items on a dirty cart and keep clean unused items on the clean carts. Disposable items are immediately thrown in the trash.

4. Reconciliation. Before transporting the carts back to CPD, the techs perform a final review and sort supplies and surgical items. A brief reconciliation occurs to determine which items are placed on the clean cart and then restocked in the CPD supermarket, and which items go to sterilization to get cleaned and then restocked in the CPD supermarket. Finally, a reconciliation report is sent to Purchasing.

5. A Purchasing Agent receives the reconciliation report which is the electronic Withdrawal Kanban indicating the items that need to be replenished from the outside supplier.

6. The Purchasing Agent submits the Supply Kanban via electronic Purchase Order for items to be replenished.

7. The Supplier receives Purchase Order from the Purchasing Agent and enters the request into an Order Fulfillment System. A Produce or "Signal" Kanban is used internally to maximize production efficiencies at the supplier.

8. Items are shipped from the outside supplier to the hospital's CPD.

9. Items from outside suppliers arrive and replenish CPD's supermarket to appropriate inventory levels.

How do you do it?

The following steps or guidelines are used to create better flow:

1. Define the target area or process that is not meeting a customer requirement, a Key Performance Indicator (KPI) or has a capacity issue.

2. Determine the type of flow method required. Understand the upstream customer's capacity and requirements.

3. Determine the flow tool that may improve the process. Understand the capacity of the process.

4. Calculate the number of Kanban Cards needed and create the Cards (if appropriate). A key factor when implementing a Pull System is the number of Kanbans Cards required. Keep in mind that these "Cards" can be electronic tallies or visual controls within various software applications. Several factors must be considered when determining the number of Kanban Cards. The key factors are:

   ❖ Average Daily Demand (ADD): What is the daily demand for the item of service?
   ❖ Lead Time (LT) of replenishment of an item or service: How long will it take to get the item or service replenished?
   ❖ Card Collection Time (CCT): How long will it take before we realize we have a pull signal?
   ❖ Safety Stock (SS): How much safety stock should be estimated for protection against from outages? Expressed as a percent, so to have 5% SS, use 1.05 for SS in the calculations.
   ❖ Container Size (CS) or standard quantity: What is the quantity or size of the product to be delivered?

These factors apply directly to a formal calculation of the number of Kanban Cards needed. The formal calculation for the number of Kanban cards is as follows:

Number of Kanban Cards = (ADD * (LT + CCT) * SS) / CS

5. Train the people who will be using the system and thoroughly explain the rules of the system.

---

6. Use the PDCA model and begin the trial. Remind people that the first attempt is a trial and to not become frustrated.

7. Follow-up to determine if modifications are needed. Initially, error on the side of too many Kanban Cards to ensure the supply of goods or services is not interrupted.

The following benefits can be obtained by creating or designing better flow:

❖ Help to stabilize process inputs and outputs
❖ Improve communications between processes
❖ Reduce wastes of delay, motion, and transport
❖ Improve overall productivity

Sensei Tips for Flow

The following are examples of flow:

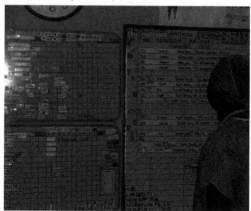

Surgical boards serve as a good example of scheduled flow.

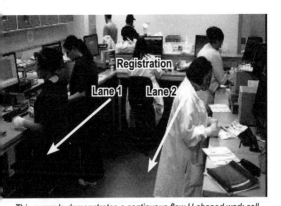

This example demonstrates a continuous flow U-shaped work cell area that distributes lab specimens to two "production" lines. The process starts for this work cell when the couriers arrive and drop off the specimens. The couriers sort and organize the specimens and then hand them to the Registration clerk. The clerk begins the initial data entry and then distributes the specimen to either Lane 1 or Lane 2. The specimen continues through the work cell to a holding rack located at the end of the line (Lane 1 or 2). At the end of the line, techs walk through the area and take the specimens to be spun at pitch increments of 10 minutes. The work is evenly distributed and the specimens are pulled through the process. Before introducing the "work cell" concept the estimated turn-around time per patient specimen was 12 hours; after the cell concept it had dropped to below 3 hours. The quality of the process was also significantly impacted, going from 5.4% defects to 0% defects! Also, with this new and improved design the numbers of specimens processed per hour worked increased from 10 per hour to 18.

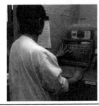

Dispensing meds is a good example of paced flow.

Improve

Quick Changeovers (QCO)

Managers will try anything easy that doesn't work
before they will try anything hard that does work.
                                    James Womack

What is it?

Quick Changeover is the ability to quickly change from delivering one product or service to delivering a completely different product or service. During delivery, providers are often required to quickly switch from delivering one product or service to delivering a completely different product or service to satisfy customer needs. The goal of QCO is to improve the customer experience by reducing waiting or delay due to changeover and adjustments. The speed in which an organization can change their delivery or service process is critical to the customer experience and overall satisfaction.

What does it do?

Quick Changeovers are a foundation for many other Lean Sigma improvements. The ability to changeover quickly affects an organization's ability to achieve Just-In-Time (JIT) deliveries, balance or level the workloads, and deliver smaller batches of customized goods or services (see the Mass Customization section for additional information). QCOs are a foundation for customer satisfaction and market dominance.

QCO improvement techniques mirror standard work methods. Use standard work tools to document and improve the changeover processes. As with standard work, the first step to reduce changeover times is to document the current state. This can be done using standard work tools of direct observation and measurement, or simple mapping tools as described earlier in this book. (Reference the Standard Work and Value Stream and Process Mapping sections for additional details on documenting the current state of a process.) Two common changeovers are hospital room changeovers and OR changeovers that can be easily improved upon.

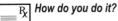

How do you do it?

The following steps or guidelines are used to implement quick changeovers:

1. Document current state.

   a. Video an equipment changeover for further analysis.
   b. Watch and study the video (laugh and/or cry).
   c. Document the activities and tasks with Standard Work Charts.
   d. Complete a Spaghetti Diagram for the changeover.

2. Separate Internal (need the machine, equipment, or process to be stopped) from External (can be done while the machine, equipment, or process is running) changeover activities.

Internal is any changeover activity or task that requires the machine, equipment, or process be stopped. Examples include: OR clean up and set-up for next surgery, notification for inpatient bed clean up by housekeeping before the patient is discharged, patient equipment need identified and requested during room assignment, etc.

External is any changeover activity or task that can be performed while the machine, equipment, or process is running. Examples include: OR housekeeping preparation, patient prep, surgeon notification, Bed Management notifies housekeeping when room is available to be cleaned after patient is discharged, etc.

3. Convert Internal to External.

   a. Prepare key items in advance of initiating changeover.
   b. Standardize functionally for supplies, tools, and equipment.
   c. Use multi-purpose supplies, tools, and equipment where possible.
   d. Consider pre-staging to speed the changeover process.
   e. Use checklists and visual systems to reduce wastes.

4. Streamline setup operations by reducing wasteful activities.

The following benefits can be obtained by implementing (or improving upon) quick changeovers:

   ❖ Improve capacity of the process
   ❖ Reduce inventories
   ❖ Reduce lead time while supporting Heijunka Leveling
   ❖ Minimize equipment downtime

Improve

🍎 Sensei Tips for Quick Changeovers

The following is an example of a surgical room quick changeover value stream map:

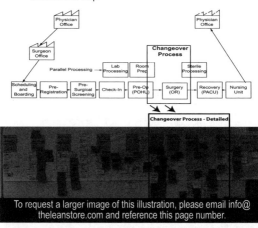

To request a larger image of this illustration, please email info@ theleanstore.com and reference this page number.

During this Perioperative Services mapping session there were 100+ wastes (dark colored Post-it Notes) identified. The team sorted the wastes into specific groups and plotted them on an Impact Map. The team decided to focus on room turn-around time for the first Kaizen Event. During the 3-day Kaizen Event the team initiated the following changes: CRNA's to notify MDAs by Spectralink when leaving POH, Recovery can assign bay during call or as they enter PACU, if there is an open bay the CRNA is to take the patient with an Anesthesia Aide to PACU, update Patient Transport via pneumatic tube system by 3 pm to level load transporters for the next day, heighten the Registration Receptionist's and Surgery's awareness of where the patient might be, e.g., on the list, in house, in ER, etc., Runner/HUC will call the Surgeon 15 minutes before scheduled surgery with status update, e.g., on-time, delayed, etc., surgical nurse to notify Housekeeping 15 minutes prior to end of surgery, reinforce SPD guidelines to surgical staff, and ensure surgical tech completes macro clean. The results were: OR turnaround time was reduced from 42 minutes to 28 minutes, along with improved patient and staff satisfaction scores, and reduced overtime.

Total Productive Maintenance (TPM)

When you are finished changing, you are finished.
Ben Franklin

What is it?

Total Productive Maintenance (TPM) refers to the tools, methods, and activities used to improve machine or equipment availability and reliability times. Hospitals have X-ray machines, telemetry equipment, lab equipment, EMR system (i.e., software updates), etc. Clearly, equipment maintenance is not just for manufacturing!

What does it do?

Organizations can reduce waste and improve their equipment effectiveness by implementing TPM practices. The overall goal of a TPM program is to reduce and eliminate equipment-related productivity losses and improve overall customer satisfaction. TPM practices involve all the people in an organization that plan, design, use, and maintain equipment and provide a system of comprehensive maintenance for the life-time of equipment.

TPM activities are designed to systematically improve the effectiveness of all equipment employed by an organization. Every person that uses equipment must have an understanding of why TPM is critical to the organization's success and thus do their part in TPM activities.

Regular inspections and audits are a part of a TPM plan. It is the PDCA process in full use as applied to equipment. Data such as Mean Time Between Failures and Mean Time to Repair can be monitored to provide improvement standards and baselines. The goal of TPM is to reduce downtime on equipment. The five main machine time losses are (1) breakdowns, setups and adjustments, (2) minor stops and waiting, (3) running defective products or creating error and rework, (4) speed losses to standards, and (5) start-up yield losses.

Improve

℞ *How do you do it?*

The following steps or guidelines are used to implement a TPM program:

1. Select equipment (primarily) or processes that are not performing to expected standards (not meeting uptime requirements, equipment not available, etc.).

2. Determine, brainstorm, and create standards for equipment maintenance. Teams often start with the machine or equipment manufactures recommendations, then make appropriate adjustments based on actual performance data.

3. Train everyone on new standards and expected responsibilities. Ensure work responsibilities are evenly distributed, if appropriate.

4. Monitor equipment and/or processes to ensure uptime has improved. Hold people accountable to complete standard work maintenance activities.

The following benefits can be obtained by implementing a TPM program:

 ❖ Improve customer satisfaction
 ❖ Improve capacity
 ❖ Reduce waste of delay
 ❖ Improve equipment reliability

Sensei Tips for Total Productive Maintenance

The following are examples of TPM:

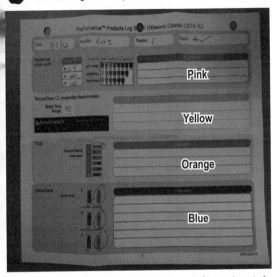

This Performance Products Log for the Ultrasonic Cleaner is part of this clinic's TPM schedule. Each of the main sections are color-coded for ease of review and completion of the evaluation (i.e., log). TPM does not have to be complicated!

Improve

Cross-Training

An organization's ability to learn, and translate that learning into action, is the ultimate competitive advantage.
Jack Welch

What is it?

Cross-training is used when one employee is required to do another employee's work. Cross-training applies to nearly every area of Lean Sigma implementations. The simplest way to manage cross-training is to complete a training matrix for the organization. The four levels of training that must be implemented for every member of the organization are:

1. Job description responsibility level
2. Improvement and problem solving tools training level
3. Next level job growth preparation level
4. Cross-training

What does it do?

The cross-training matrix is the road map for employee development and improved work efficiency. To complete the cross-training matrix, first identify individual job description, Knowledge, Skill, and Ability (KS&A) requirements, and document them in the Job Description section of the training matrix form. Identify improvement and problem solving KS&A requirements. Consider the following core training areas:

- ❖ Business KS&A
- ❖ Technical KS&A
- ❖ People KS&A

| $\boxed{R_x}$ | ***How do you do it?*** |

The following steps or guidelines are used to implement cross- training:

1. Identify and list all employees in a table.

2. Complete training needs assessment for each employee based on each employee's job description/ current work duties and back-up responsibilities, as well as any future development needs. Place the specific training needs in a table to establish the training matrix.

3. Identify the current level of proficiency or competence in the matrix for every employee.

4. Identify gaps or training needs for each employee and the organization.

5. Develop a training plan based on the gaps identified in the training matrix and time line for delivery.

6. Update the matrix as progress is made.

7. Repeat this process periodically (at least annually).

The following benefits can be obtained by implementing a cross-training program:

- ❖ Break up the monotony of the week
- ❖ Reduce work intensity of the RN staff, providing more time for direct patient care
- ❖ Create teamwork to understand how the total process or value stream works
- ❖ Allow the manager to discover which workers are well suited for different positions
- ❖ Help patients to get billing question answered on first call due to more people having the answer (solve problem on first call)
- ❖ Allow for easier filling-in for staff emergencies and vacations
- ❖ Improve process' or departments' capacity
- ❖ Allow organizational knowledge to be shared

Improve

Sensei Tips for Cross-Training

The following is an example of a cross-training matrix:

Employee	Job Title	Coordinating with Insurance Companies	Billing and Insurance Claims	Scheduling	Computer Skills	Patient Care Coordinating	Telephone Skills	Time Management
		Key Process Duties						
3423	44	1	2	1	3	3	3	4
3456	33	3	1	3	1	3	3	3
3954	11	2	2	3	1	4	3	3
1896	33	3	3	4	4	4	4	3
4389	07	2	3	3	3	3	1	3
4574	07	3	3	3	1	3	3	3

44 - Clinic - Admin. Assistant - Front Desk
33 - Clinic - Business Office Associate - Billing
11 - Clinic - Front Office Manager
07 - Clinic - Medical Receptionist

Legend: 1 = Initial training
2 = Developing
3 = Proficient
4 = Trainer

This Cross-Training Matrix shows the training for each employee at a small Urology clinic.

Lean Thinking Statements for the Improve Phase

The following Lean Thinking Statement assessment should be done as an individual and, if desired, combined and discussed as a team. If the team leader realizes that many of the items are an issue for certain team members, then maybe a one-on-one with those specific individuals would be appropriate. Or, if a few of the team members have similar concerns over one or two of the statements, then possibly these should be addressed with the team. Continue with open and honest dialogue with the team. As a team member, it is YOUR responsibility to address any of the statements that hinder YOUR individual input to the team's progress. These statements are not to be taken lightly!

Use the 5 Level Likert Scale for the following statements:

> 1 - Strongly Disagree
> 2 - Disagree
> 3 - Neither Agree nor Disagree
> 4 - Agree
> 5 - Strongly Agree

I understand the Lean tools being applied. _____
I participated in adapting the Lean tools in our project. _____
I understand the value of standard work. _____
I believe 5S is useful Lean tool that can and will be used at some point in the implementation. _____
The future state map was helpful in being our road map. _____
I can contribute to this team. _____
I am confident in discussing this project with my colleagues. _____
I see the value in this team's approach. _____
I believe I can add value to this team. _____
I believe my ideas will be heard and considered. _____

Total Score: [   ]

If your score is less than 80% (40 points), then more work should be completed before moving on to the Control Phase. Ensure the A3 Project Report Sections 5. Future State, 6. Implementation Plan, and 7. Verify Results are nearly completed.

Improve

Notes

The Control Phase

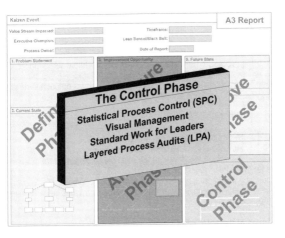

The Control Phase

Statistical Process Control (SPC)
Visual Management
Standard Work for Leaders
Layered Process Audits (LPA)

Tools listed in this section are most likely to be used at this time. All the tools can be applicable at any phase of a Kaizen Project as determined by the needs of the project team.

Statistical Process Control (SPC)

It's not the numbers that make a process, rather than it's the process that should make the numbers.

Unknown

What is it?

Statistical Process Control *is used to monitor and control process outputs.* SPC monitors processes to determine if they are in control, are developing trends, and know when they go out of control. Processes are said to be in control if only natural or common cause variation occurs. SPC Charts, also referred to as Control or Shewhart Charts, identify when special cause variation has entered into the process. They are used to predict the future performance of a process. If special cause variation has entered into the process, additional actions are required to contain the process output and regain control. SPC methods are very powerful in the Control Phase.

What does it do?

SPC Charts work with two types of data: variable data and attribute data. **Variable data** *measures along a continuous scale for length, time, or weight, for example.* **Attribute data** *assumes only two values (good or bad, pass or fail, etc.) and is measured by counting the frequency of items matching the condition.* The following SPC Charting techniques are used for the data types and sampling abilities specified.

Types of Variable Data Charts

❖ Run Chart: Numerous applications (covered in the Diagnosis Phase)
❖ X and Moving Range Chart: Where the sample size is 1
❖ X-Bar and Range (R) Chart: Where the sample size is 3 - 7, evaluating the cycle time of a process
❖ X-Bar and S Chart: Where the sample size is >10, such as when measuring the time of each transaction completed during a day's activities

---

Types of Attribute Data Charts

- ❖ Use a P Chart (Percent Error Rate or non-conforming) to measure the number of transactions with errors versus total transactions processed
- ❖ Use a C Chart (Defects per unit) to measure the number of errors on specific transactions

Control Charts for variables, such as X and Moving Range, X-Bar and R Charts, and X-Bar and S Charts, are developed by taking a number of samples (usually 25 - 30 samples) of a certain size (usually 3 - 10 items per sample) from a process all thought to be in statistical control, and calculating the sample means and ranges. Using standard statistical methods, the grand mean (or mean of the sample means) and average range (R-Bar) are calculated and used as center lines for the segments of the X-Bar and R Charts.

Establish control limits for the sample X-Bar and R values. Then the sample values are plotted on their respective charts. Any values or groups of values are deemed to be out-of-control if any of the following conditions occur:

- ❖ One point above the Upper Control Limit (UCL)
- ❖ One point below the Lower Control Limit (LCL)
- ❖ Any increasing run or trend of seven consecutive points
- ❖ Any decreasing run or trend of seven consecutive points
- ❖ Seven consecutive points above the X-bar
- ❖ Seven consecutive points below the X-bar
- ❖ Any point outside the range control limits
- ❖ Two out of three consecutive points in the outer one-third region of the control limits
- ❖ Four out of five points in the outer two-thirds region of the control limits

Determine assignable causes for any out of control condition. The out-of-control samples (if applicable) must be discarded, and the Control Chart characteristics must be re-calculated. Additional tools, such as brainstorming, 5 Why Analysis, etc. can be used to determine the out-of-control condition and what must be done to correct it. Similar processes are used to calculate sample statistics and control limits for attribute charts.

Control

---

3 Standard Deviations (3 SD or 3 sigma) gives a "confidence level" which includes 99.73% of all events or 99.73% of ALL random and similar events will fall within +/- 3 SD. X-Bar plus 3 SD, referred to as the UCL, is the + 3 SD marker and X-Bar minus 3 SD, referred to as the LCL, is the -3 SD marker. This is used to recognize what is "normal" and what is "abnormal." Basically, as long as the individual plots are between the UCL and the LCL, the process is exhibiting "NORMAL" variation. However, 99.73% of events means that 0.27% of the points on the Control Chart would be outside the +/-3 SD control limits when the process is operating in control, and these would be false signals.

For very critical processes, it is recommended to use +/- 1SD. This most likely would result in many false signals, but there would also be very few missed signals. This would provide increased protection against the process producing an error.

How do you do it?

The following steps or guidelines are used to initiate Statistical Process Control:

1. Determine the measurement method by choosing the data to collect and the category of control chart to use: variable or attribute. Use variable data whenever possible because it provides higher quality information - it does not rely on sometimes arbitrary distinctions between good and bad, pass or fail, etc.

2. Qualify the measurement system by using some form of Measurement System Analysis (MSA). *MSA evaluates the test methods, measuring instruments, and the entire process of obtaining measurements to ensure the integrity of data used for analysis (usually quality analysis). This helps to communicate the implications of measurement error for decisions made about a product or process.*

3. Initiate data collection and SPC charting by developing a plan to collect data in a random fashion at a determined frequency. Train the data collectors in proper measurement and charting techniques.

4. Develop and document a reaction plan by creating a defined plan to guide the actions of those using the chart in the event of an out-of-control or out-of-specification condition.

5. Add the SPC chart to the Control Plan. A **Control Plan** is a centralized document that tracks the measurement method and control of all significant process characteristics of a process or product.

6. Collect relevant data; calculate and plot control limits after 20 - 25 subgroups.

7. Determine if the process is in control (i.e., statistically stable over time). The determination is made by observing the plot point patterns and determines if there are any out-of-process events occurring.

8. Continually analyze charts to identify root cause(s).

9. Design and implement actions to eliminate root causes that are responsible for the out-of-control condition.

10. Periodically calculate Cp and Cpk and compare to benchmark.

Note: Consult a statistics book to further learn about Cp, Cpk, and process stability.

The following benefits can be obtained by using Statistical Process Control:

  ❖ Optimize information needed for decision-making
  ❖ Provide understanding of business baselines, insights for improvements, and communication of value and results of processes
  ❖ Provide real-time analysis to establish controllable process baselines
  ❖ Allow for decision-making based on facts

Note: Consider using the Pivot Table function of Excel with Control Charts to thoroughly analyze process characteristics. Further analysis, if out-of-control conditions occur, can then utilize Fishbone Diagrams and Root Cause (or 5 Why) Analysis.

Control

Sensei Tips for Statistical Process Control

The following SPC Charts shows various levels of control:

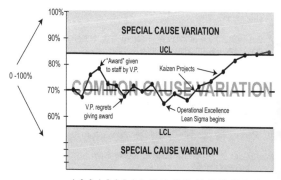

This hospital's SPC Control Chart is for the question "I would recommend this hospital and clinic to others." from the NCR Picket Patient Satisfaction Survey. Prior to a implementing Operational Excellence (a Lean Sigma program), the V.P. had prematurely given awards to staff due to the improvements in scores (not remembering that this was most likely due to common cause variation). Upon initiating a formal program and completing a few Kaizen Events, there was a significant improvement in the scores. This example clearly shows that prior to understanding Lean Sigma (and specifically Control Charts) managers had led by innuendos and rumors, not by statistical data. As the trend continued, the Upper and Lower Control Limits were recalculated.

Visual Management

Create a work environment that is self-explaining,
self-regulating, and self-improving – where what is
suppose to happen does happen, on-time, every time.
Gwendolyn Galsworth

What is it?

Visual Management is the use of visual techniques that
graphically display relevant business performance data.
The relevant business performance data can be Key Performance
Indicators (KPIs), customer mandates, governmental compliances, etc.

What is it?

Visual Management is a higher-level approach to visual controls
used to monitor an organization's, a work team's, or an individual's
performance. Visual management techniques can be very powerful
drivers in leading organizations through Lean Sigma transformations.
Visual management techniques include visual displays such as
Performance Dashboards, Visual Management Boards, Storyboards,
Hoshin Planning, A3s, or other means by which performance is closely
monitored and displayed. These can help people quickly see and
understand any current and future states of an organization. (The A3
was described on pages 31 - 37.)

Hoshin Planning

Hoshin Planning is a method to capture the strategic goals of
the organization and systematically cascade them throughout the
organization in a highly defined and specified method. Hoshin planning
utilizes a participative process to communicate and clarify the strategic
goals to all levels of an organization. This process captures flashes of
insight about the future and brings the appropriate resources together to
make them a reality. Hoshin Planning is one of many Policy Deployment
techniques, and is the preferred method for Lean Sigma organizations.

Hoshin Planning is designed to use the collective thinking of all employees
to make their organization the best in its field. It is the process of setting
goals throughout the organization based on the strategic goals and top
managers and middle managers must be bold enough to delegate to

employees working the processes as much authority as possible to meeting those goals. The result of this process is to have daily, or more frequent measurable control activities linked to the company strategy.

Hoshin Planning provides the following benefits:

❖ Allow for a shared goal focus with employee involvement
❖ Provide for a common communication platform that all employees can relate to
❖ Provide accountability to daily activities through measurements

The following PDCA cycle is the core principle of Hoshin Planning:

PLAN
1. WHO will be the lead from each of the cross-functional areas?
2. WHAT bold objectives are facing the organization?
3. WHEN are the start and finish dates of each action item?
4. HOW are the objectives tied to the strategic direction?
5. HOW do we proceed, by WHICH sub-actions to move us along?
6. WHAT are the measurements that are tied to the success of the organization as a whole?
7. WHAT resources can be applied to the objectives?
8. HOW OFTEN is there a cross-functional team review?

DO
1. DO the items that are part of the PLAN phase.

CHECK
1. MEASURE the actual results achieved.
2. COMPARE the Year-To-Date target # that was set in the PLAN phase.
3. EVALUATE the measurements.
4. ANALYZE variation between actual results and target expectations. Use Quality Improvement tools (i.e., Check Sheet, Run Chart, Histogram, Pareto Diagram, Flow Chart or Process Map, Fishbone Diagram, and Control Chart) for further investigation and root cause analysis.

ACT
1. TAKE CORRECTIVE ACTION to get back on track.
2. VERIFY corrective action frequently.

The PDCA phases or cycle repeats itself on an annual basis. Employee engagement will drive its successful deployment.

Performance Dashboards

A **Performance Dashboard** is a visual aid that translates the organization's strategy into objectives, metrics, initiatives, and tasks customized to each group and individual in an organization. It further enables management to measure, monitor, and manage the key activities and processes needed to achieve their goals as well as make critical business decisions more quickly. Many times a Dashboard will include or reference the Key Performance Indicators (KPIs) or parts of the Balanced Scorecard of the organization.

Dashboards have long been a fixture in automobiles and other vehicles and only in the last 20 years or so have organizations adopted their usage. In business, these Dashboards initially started out as Executive Information Systems (EIS), but they never gained a foothold through an organization because they were geared to so few people in each company and were cumbersome to change due to Information Technology dependencies. Since Information Technology has advanced at such a rapid pace, supplanted by the Web as the preeminent platform for running applications and delivering information, Dashboards have evolved into an everyday business improvement tool known as a Performance Dashboard. Furthermore, with the use of Open Source applications, organizations can now create effective Performance Dashboards on their own, using their existing software tools and applications.

Dashboards may or may not be balanced. If balanced, they are referred to as Balanced Scorecards. **Balanced Scorecards** are a form of performance management that is used by managers to keep track of the activities of the organization to control and monitor key financial and non-financial metrics, typically no more than about 20. The three areas of 'balance' to consider are metric-to-metric balance, leading and lagging balance, and area-to-area balance. There is said to be metric-to-metric balance to Performance Dashboards if the performance measures provide protection from optimization of one performance goal at the expense of another. For example, an organization could improve (or decrease) their patient wait time by adding more staff. This may be good for the patient wait time, but bad for profitability. A measure of total patient wait time per staff member would need to be tracked to "balance" the measures.

Control

Another concept of 'balance' is to have leading and lagging performance measures. A leading indicator to patient satisfaction may be employee attendance. If employees do not show up at work when required, patient satisfaction (a lagging or after the service measure) may suffer. Typically, good people performance leads to good operational performance, which leads to good patient/customer satisfaction performance, which leads to good financial performance. There is a causal relationship between people, operations, customer/patient satisfaction, and financial performance, and it is important to have balance in measures in these areas.

The last area to consider is area-to-area balance within an organization. Since work flows horizontally through organizations, it is critical to seek balance by measuring indicators in each area of an organization. Organizations should seek balanced Performance Dashboards in the key areas of operations (operational productivity, quality, and growth), revenue, and innovation or new service offerings.

There are numerous commercial Performance Dashboard applications available, with many offering a 30-day free trial. If what you require is not too complicated or involved, consider using Microsoft Excel or other applications within your current system to display the information that is required.

Visual Management Board

*A **Visual Management Board** (or **Status-At-A-Glance Board**) is a visual aid that has the typical headings of Safety, Quality, Cost (or Savings), Delivery and People to reflect current measurements as well as problem solving or continuous improvement activities.* They are designed to engage employees and leaders visiting the area. They are simple and easy to read and are tailored to the department.

A Visual Management Board provides the following:

- ❖ The status (real-time, hourly, or daily) of the area or process
- ❖ A quick way to determine if the area or process is meeting its goal, and if not, what steps (countermeasures or improvements) are being taken
- ❖ Measurements that include goals/targets (expected) and actual results
- ❖ Evidence that the information is maintained and current
- ❖ The key people involved in the process (may be a listing of all employees working the area, may be a picture of the Employee of the Week, may be team photo of the current improvement team, etc.)

A Visual Management Board is designed by creating distinct areas of an appropriately sized bulletin board. The first or main area, Performance Measures, should reflect the key performance indicators for the specific area or process (i.e., Patient Satisfaction, Quality, Safety, etc. for healthcare) with appropriate charts and graphs. If appropriate, have photos of the employees also on the board. The major (or second) area of the board should include the following four sections (1) Kaizen Project defined: the issue or problem clearly defined relative to a Performance Measure, (2) History/Analysis: this could be a value stream or process map, Fishbone Diagram, 5 Why Analysis, Pareto Chart, etc., (3) PDCAs, Countermeasures or Improvement Activities: this could be an Action Item List detailing the specific process changes, and (4) Results: this could be a completed A3 Project Report or any other appropriate charts or graphs.

When representing a time line or schedule from the A3 Report (implementation or Kaizen activities) or if you are using some other project management tool, consider color-coding the activities for easy of viewing. For example, tasks or activities can be listed in black, deliverables can be green, and on schedule, and red can indicate behind schedule.

Storyboards

*The **Storyboard** is a poster-size or larger framework for displaying all the key information from the Lean Sigma project.* It also is a version of the A3 for problem solving. It can be created in Excel, Visio, or some other application. The Storyboard is organized into various areas that can be represented by a graph, illustration, and/or a simple sentence or two. The information is then displayed on a format that is graphically rich and engaging. The Storyboard will display many of the tools used throughout the project.

The Storyboard segments may include some, if not all, of the following categories:

- ❖ Reason for Selecting the Project (Problem Statement)
- ❖ Data Chart of Present Condition (Pareto Chart, Fishbone, etc.)
- ❖ Target Goal
- ❖ Plan of Action (portion of Gantt Chart)
- ❖ Results (New Standards, Metrics, etc.)
- ❖ Team Recognition
- ❖ Next Target

The Storyboard should be posted in an area where the continuous improvement activities occur and should be updated as new information is obtained. Storyboards can be fun in design, many times taking on a graphical theme (e.g., an Emergency department in a hospital may display the various sections in comparison to an ambulance, an Operating Room comparison to an operating table, the billing department to various currency denominations, etc.). Team members responsible for creating the Storyboard should make it engaging and use creativity by using color, themes, etc.

In today's fast paced global marketplace, Storyboarding techniques are becoming more virtual, meaning that rather than a large board displayed in a specific area, Lean Sigma improvement teams create Storyboards that can be accessed on the Web.

Note: The A3 (the 11" x 17" paper size) is often used to represent the Hoshin Plan with "telling the story." It can be also be used for displaying a Storyboard or problem solving project as well as be the framework for conducting and documenting a Kaizen Event.

Yokoten

Yokoten means *"best practice sharing"* or *"taking from one place to another."* It encompasses the methods of communicating, documenting, and distributing knowledge horizontally within an organization (peer-to-peer) about what worked and what did not work from an improvement project.

Yokoten is a form of knowledge management. At its most basic level, Yokoten is the set of documents a team keeps as a history of the problems/solutions encountered. Yokoten can also be the library of A3 problem reports (Storyboards) that a team or work group maintains for everyone to access. As a knowledge management device, the Yokoten process ensures information becomes part of the organizational knowledge base. At Toyota, there is an expectation that copying a good idea will be followed by some added "kaizen" to that idea (copy + kaizen = yokoten).

Yokoten standardizes the documentation of a solution and shares it. This sharing of standards and/or best practice procedures across an organization promotes employee development and organizational learning. Do not underestimate the importance of this.

| R_X | *How do you do it?*

The following steps or guidelines are used to adopt visual management techniques:

1. Create a team of employees from the work areas that visual management techniques will use.

2. Determine for each process or area what information is needed to do the work properly.

3. Determine how to measure success of people, timeliness, quality, productivity, customer, and financial.

4. Determine appropriate connection points in upstream and downstream processes.

5. Develop innovative, creative, and visually compelling methods to share and communicate vital information upstream and downstream.

6. Standardize visual management techniques to drive continuous improvement activities.

The following benefits can be obtained by using visual management techniques:

❖ Lead to information sharing and better decision-making
❖ Allow managers to make decisions more accurately and efficiently
❖ Align and support Balance Scorecard metrics
❖ Support elimination of waste
❖ Allow for quick-response to issues and problems
❖ Assist to maintain or sustain continuous improvement activities
❖ Communicate needed information to the right people
❖ Instill the message, "what gets measured, gets done"
❖ Allow for a single vision of what is required
❖ Empower employees with self-service access to information
❖ Increase coordination between departments
❖ Allow workers to take ownership of their performance-to-target goals and eliminate the need for management to micro-manage

---

🍎 *Sensei Tips for Visual Management*

The following are examples of visual management:

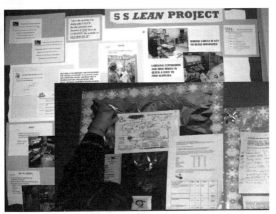

These are examples of storyboards from two hospital's improvement teams conveying their improvement projects.

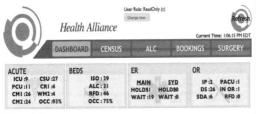

This is an example of a Performance Dashboard that uses good visuals to display relevant information.

Yokoten Worksheet

Problem: Delays in moving patient from ED at time of disposition to arrival in their hospital bed (unit)

Presentation Date: July 2nd

List team members that will present at Yokoten meeting.	Convey pre and post measurements in simple form.
Margaret Rodriguez and Sue Richards	Patient Satisfaction: Pre – avg 2.3 Post – avg 3.9 Cycle time, Dispo-to-Admit: Pre – avg 170 mins Post – avg 102 mins (-68 min)

Place a checkmark (✓) by each waste that was eliminated.

	Overproduction		Overprocessing
✓	Waiting (Queues)		Inventory
✓	Motion	✓	Defects
	Transport	✓	People's Skills

Convey timeline in simple bar graph form.

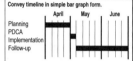

	April	May	June
Planning			
PDCA			
Implementation			
Follow-up			

Place a checkmark (✓) by the tools used. Identify the main tools used by placing a circle around each checkmark.

⊘ 5S		✓ Effective Meetings		✓ Idea Kaizen		✓ Perf. Measurement		✓ Takt Time
✓ 5 Why Analysis		⊘ Effective Team		✓ Impact Map		Pitch		✓ Training Plan
✓ Accepting Change		⊘ Failure Prevention		Just-In-Time		✓ Problem ID		⊘ Value Stream Map
✓ Brainstorming		⊘ Fishbone		✓ Kanban		✓ Pull Systems		⊘ VOC
✓ Continuous Flow		✓ Flowchart		⊘ Mistake Proofing		✓ Run Chart		✓ Waste Audit
✓ Cycle Time		✓ Gantt Chart		✓ Pareto Diagram		Runners		⊘ Work Load Balancing
✓ Data Collection		✓ Heijunka - Leveling		✓ Paynter Chart		⊘ Standard Work		Yokoten

List any Idea Kaizens that were generated.	List recommendations to management.
1. Move printers from under counter for ED clerk 2. Change lab printer to green paper for easy ID of lab results	1. Have Mgt attend monthly ED department meetings to ensure that communication continues 2. Continue working with Bed Control, Housekeeping, and Units to promote bed readiness

List a few experiences regarding the team process.	List recommendations to other teams.
1. Initial meetings were difficult due to different perceptions and expectations of team members 2. Group development of the detailed value stream, and collection of data, helped team to move forward toward solutions	1. Need a cross-functional team including front line staff, supervisors, and downstream customers in the process 2. Allow team to come together through group exercises 3. Make sure to allow stakeholders a chance to give feedback on proposed solutions, prior to implementation

List overall benefits from the PDCA Kaizen Event.	List contact person and email for additional info.
1. Patients feel as if hospital wants to admit them – reflected in overall satisfaction scores 2. Staff feels less stressed in this portion of the work – easier to "get things done" 3. Physicians like the improved communication among staff	Sue Richards, Team Facilitator, 586-441-2244 sue.richards@oakviewhosp.org Margaret Rodriguez, Process Owner 586-441-3426 margaret.rodriguez@oakviewhosp.org

The location of the electronic version of the Yokoten, as well as the supporting materials, can be found at:

http://www.oakvalley.oakviewhosp.org/yokoten/EDAdmit_Oakview

This is an example of a Yokoten. The improvement team did a good job in identifying the main wastes, applying Lean Sigma tools, and achieving significant results.

Visual Management Board

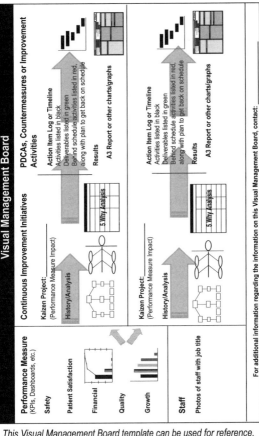

Performance Measure (KPIs, Dashboards, etc.)	Continuous Improvement Initiatives	PDCAs, Countermeasures or Improvement Activities

Performance Measure (KPIs, Dashboards, etc.)

Safety

Patient Satisfaction

Financial

Quality

Growth

Staff

Photos of staff with job title

Continuous Improvement Initiatives

Kaizen Project:
(Performance Measure Impact)

History/Analysis

5 Why Analysis

PDCAs, Countermeasures or Improvement Activities

Action Item Log or Timeline
Activities listed in black
Deliverables listed in green
Behind schedule activities listed in red, along with plan to get back on schedule

Results

A3 Report or other charts/graphs

For additional information regarding the information on this Visual Management Board, contact: _____

This Visual Management Board template can be used for reference. Ensure your Board is simple to view and understand, accessible for staff and management, current, and has a standardized format when compared to other departments.

Control

Standard Work for Leaders

*A leader is one who knows the way, goes the way,
and shows the way.*
John C. Maxwell

What is it?

Standard Work for Leaders prescribes specific tasks,
actions, and time frames for completion of work for a
manager or supervisor. Standard Work for Leaders is a concept derived
from general standard work practices to follow. Every position in every
organization should have standard work processes. This can also be
referred to as leadership behaviors and methods.

What does it do?

Standard Work for Leaders is critical on several levels. First,
standard work is the basic building block for continuous
improvement. Without standard work for everyone, there is no
baseline for improvement efforts, and improvements cannot be properly
documented and measured. Leaders need to be responsible and
accountable to continually improve their personal effectiveness.

Second, Standard Work for Leaders assists leaders to understand how
the organization, teams, and individuals perform and address areas
of low performance. Standard Work for Leaders involves monitoring
the Key Performance Indicators (KPIs) of the organization and taking
corrective and preventative action as required. This is critical to an
organization's sustained success.

Additionally, as improvement teams see leaders performing standard
work teams will better understand that standard work for their positions
is here to stay. The best way to show people that the organization is
serious about implementing Lean Sigma methods and tools is for leaders
to practice the methods and tools themselves. By "walking the talk,"
leaders also build trust with workers. Trust is another key ingredient for
sustained Lean Sigma success.

Standard Work for Leaders defines, for every level leader, a systematic approach to setting the direction for the organization and deploying the tactical plan to achieve goals. This includes defining Key Performance Indicators and targets, identifying improvement target areas, team building, teaching, or communicating. Standard Work for Leaders defines a systematic approach to running a world-class organization and allows a clear and standard method of back-up or support when a leader is unavailable.

How do you do it?

The following steps or guidelines are used to create Standard Work for Leaders for your organization:

Note: See example on pages 220 - 223.

1. Create a table of the main functional levels within the organization.

2. Ensure all job descriptions are up-to-date.

3. Create and ensure each functional level of the organization understands and has relevant measurements available.

4. Create a list for frequency of review for the measurements of each functional level (i.e., daily, monthly, quarterly, etc.).

5. Determine frequency of meetings to review measurements for each functional level.

6. Create and communicate action plans to address areas of concern or problems.

The following benefits can be obtained by creating and using Standard Work for Leaders:

❖ Lead to information sharing and better decision-making
❖ Support better communication
❖ Build trust among the work group
❖ Improve alignment from organizational goals to departmental or work group goals

The table which follows describes typical Standard Work for Leaders at various levels in an organization. It provides a general guideline on what is expected at each level. Use this as a guide when establishing Standard Work for Leaders within your organization.

Activity and Frequency

Level	Daily	Weekly
	Promote and conduct activities to meet the strategic direction of the organization. Lead by example!	Establish rolling weekly agendas and conduct weekly meetings with each departmental manager. Use the DMAIC, process and project management format. Meeting should focus on KPIs and on-going improvement initiatives.
Corporate Leader	Review and analyze required corporate productivity reports. Meet with appropriate departmental managers to review reports. Acknowledge success.	Track requirements from what was discussed and expected at weekly meetings.
	Focus on reports that show a negative trend. Gather data and conduct appropriate meetings. Communicate once per day to all direct reports demonstrating engagement and involvement.	Continue to monitor KPIs that show a negative trend. Continue to work to support improvement efforts.

Activity and Frequency

Monthly	Semi-Annually	Annually
Establish rolling monthly agenda and conduct monthly meetings with departmental managers.	Review all organizational level KPIs, goals, and individual subordinate performance measurements. Check for alignment with organizational strategy. Modify as needed.	Review all organizational level KPIs, goals, and individual subordinate performance measurements. Check for alignment with organizational strategy. Modify as needed.
	Provide mini-performance feedback sessions for each direct report. Assign appropriate improvement plans to ensure employee development and KPIs are met, as applicable.	Conduct performance appraisals for each direct report. Assign appropriate improvement plans to ensure employee development and KPIs are met, as applicable.
		Review strategic direction, adjust to market conditions, and develop alignment with new or revised KPIs.

Control

Activity and Frequency

Level	Daily	Weekly
	Follow appropriate work instructions, procedures, and complete Job Description activities. Lead by example!	Establish and conduct weekly meetings with supervisors and team leaders.
Departmental Manager or Supervisor	Complete and analyze departmental productivity reports. Meet with appropriate leads to review reports. Acknowledge success.	Be available for direct reports for contact.
	Establish pro-active actions to address any and all negative trends. Initiate Lean Sigma teams for appropriate issues. Look for other continuous improvement activities.	Monitor all performance measurements and follow-up with teams or individuals that have responsibility to address negative trends.
	Follow appropriate work instructions, procedures, and complete Job Description activities. Lead by example!	Establish and conduct weekly meetings for continuous improvement efforts.
Work Team Leader	Complete daily tasks, encourage improvement initiatives, support departmental initiatives, and acknowledge workers that contribute ideas.	Be attentive to employee's concerns (and ideas for improvement).

Activity and Frequency

Monthly	Semi-Annually	Annually
Review monthly departmental goals or KPIs with team leader and employees, if appropriate.	Communicate the organizations priorities including customer satisfaction.	Create and implement an innovative communication plan to clearly define to organization members the vision and mission that includes customer satisfaction.
Continue to support continuous improvement and problem solving teams.	Communicate progress to date to all employees. Continue to support continuous improvement efforts.	Continue to address departmental areas of concern and allocate appropriate resources to ensure success.

Monthly	Semi-Annually	Annually
Review monthly goals with employees, if appropriate.	Communicate the organizations priorities including customer satisfaction to all employees.	Create and implement an innovative communication plan to clearly define to organization members the vision and mission that includes customer satisfaction.
Continue to demonstrate support and enthusiasm for continuous improvement efforts.	Provide employees with specific improvement initiatives that have contributed to improving departmental measures.	Continue to work to develop employees.

Control

Sensei Tips for Standard Work for Leaders

The following is an example of how one intact work team stan dardized their daily meetings for their leaders:

Seattle Grace Team Huddle Process Standard Tool

Huddles are intended as a method to communicate with our associates and listen to their voice; focusing on the critical success factors of patient safety, patient experience, and financial stewardship while soliciting improvement opportunities. Huddles are to be held with all of your associates at a designated time and on every shift. Those departments with only 1 associate or if there is only 1 associate on duty, such as 2nd and 3rd shifts, combine those associates into your morning or evening Huddle.

The Department Manager is responsible to ensure the Huddles are following a standardize Work Sequence (see below). The Manager will conduct the huddle(s) or assign a facilitator to conduct the Huddle(s) when the Manager cannot be present.

Issues that cannot be resolved by a leader should be communicated up to the next level of the department leadership.

Discuss the ground rules: Time is limited to 15 minutes or less (with a timekeeper), issues or problems identified are only reviewed at this time (unless there are quick and easy solutions)

Description of Work Sequence	Time	Critical Points
Step 1: Reflection/Story/Thought (of the day)	0.5	Welcome everyone.
Step 2: General Departmental Announcements and Recognition	1.5	Discuss any wins, celebrations, appreciations, etc.
Step 3: Review Safety Issues *Any issues related to patient or associate safety.*	2.0	Address all issues identified, those that require escalation or serious safety events, bring to Leadership Huddle.
Step 4: Review Equipment Issues *Any equipment issues (missing, lost, broken) that may hinder you from doing your job.*	1.0	Address all issues identified, and those that require additional work orders should be offline from the Huddle.
Step 5: Review Patient Experience Issues *Any patient that wouldn't rate us as an "always" meeting their expectations.*	2.0	Address all issues identified, those that require additional escalation, bring to Leadership Huddle.
Step 6: Identify Throughput Issues	1.0	Identify any barriers to discharges. Bring information to daily Bed Huddle.
Step 7: Matrix Review #1 *Review daily progress of 3 or less items.*	2.0	Review metrics from previous day. If progress is not being made, discuss the barriers preventing the team from achieving the goal. If meeting the goal, discuss what is going well.
Step 8: Real-Time Rounding Feedback	2.0	Review metrics from previous day. If progress is not being made, discuss the barriers preventing the team from achieving the goal. If meeting the goal, discuss what is going well.
Step 9: Daily Buzz	1.0	Ask what are you hearing about the units and throughout the house.
Step 10:Closing Comments	1.0	Thank everyone for attending!

This example was Standard Work for Leaders for Floor Managers. It allowed (1) an awareness of "what's going on" in the area (2) a chance to plan your and your team's day, (3) early problem identification and resolution of issues, and (4) an opportunity to gather information to "communicate up."

Layered Process Audits (LPA)

A foolproof system is no match for a system-proof fool!
Anonymous

What is it?

Layered Process Audits (LPA) is a system of process audits performed by multiple levels of workers, supervisors, and managers to monitor key process characteristics and verify process conformance on an ongoing basis. LPAs ensure that standard work methods are used and that processes are performing as expected to desired outcomes.

What does it do?

Typically, a Layered Process Auditing system is based on a series of process audits for critical or high risk processes, multiple layers of audits by workers, supervisors and managers from different areas, and a system of reporting and follow-up that ensures conformance and, when warranted, corrective actions are implemented. Layered Process Audits provide an excellent tool for sustaining improvements in processes. LPAs help organizations error-proof their processes/systems.

To get the most out of an LPA system, perform real-time audits. An audit performed on last week's work may be revealing, but will not provide the opportunity for avoiding problems, only fixing them in hindsight. An audit performed as is being completed affords the worker the opportunity to correct undesirable behaviors real-time.

Conducting the LPAs are usually based on the volume or level of risk associated with the process or action. Real-time audits are often used in the healthcare area where a patient may be asked several times to confirm who they are, the issue or area of the pending surgery or procedure, etc. This type of repetitive real-time audit is sometimes called a redundant check if the LPA is not documented. Redundant checks are often helpful where there is a great deal of human interaction in the process, and there is a great potential risk if the process is done wrong.

Control

Another area where redundancy checks are commonly used is in the cockpit of airplanes before the flight begins. The pilot and co-pilot complete redundancy checks on operating systems of aircraft, as well as function checks of other issues concerning the flight.

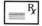 *How do you do it?*

The following steps or guidelines are used for creating and implementing a Layered Process Audit system:

1. Understand the following four elements that comprise an effective Layered Process Audit system:

   a. A Collection or Series of Audits - Audits are simply an organized group of questions designed to examine equipment, supplies, or a process. Audits in an LPA system should focus on areas where errors represent a high-risk for customers and organizations.
   b. Layers of Auditors - In an LPA system, your collection of audits is performed on a scheduled basis, at a predetermined frequency, by multiple layers of management from across the organization.
   c. Prevention and Containment - For a Layered Process Audit system to be truly effective, it must integrate analysis, action, and improvements. If an auditor finds a non-conformance while performing an audit, that auditor should not only record their finding, but also take immediate initial corrective action to ensure customers are not affected by the potential error.
   d. Reporting and Follow-up - Information about the finding should be recorded and readily available to management for later analysis. Use regular management reviews to ensure the effectiveness of the LPA system.

2. Understand the following audit types of LPAs. Each type of audit can be performed to a published schedule or conducted by surprise.

   a. Simple audit – This is a simple yes or no question and answer format to determine if the process is working properly and may be performed concurrent or after the process is complete.
   b. Concurrent audit – This LPA is completed as the process is being delivered to ensure completeness, accuracy, and/or customer satisfaction.
   c. Layered audit - This is an audit by a different level of leadership to ensure the LPAs are being performed to plan.
   d. Self-audit – This is an audit completed by the worker providing the service or working the process. This audit is basically a checklist to ensure the process is complete and accurate, and that the customer is satisfied.
   e. Co-worker Audit – This is similar to a Self-audit, but it is completed by a co-worker or peer.
   f. Internal audits – to verify that current policies and procedures are in keeping with the current operating environment or conditions

3. Develop a layered process audit form and specify the items, who will perform the audit, and the frequency of audit.

4. Perform audits to the plan, post visually, and monitor audit system outputs and results.

5. Take corrective and preventative actions as necessary.

The following benefits can be obtained by using a Layered Process Audit system:

   ❖ Drive desired behavior
   ❖ Allow for critical review of processes
   ❖ Ensure employee, supervisor, and manager engagement
   ❖ Bring problems to light early on
   ❖ Improve the quality of the product or service
   ❖ Keep everyone focused on the process characteristics

Control

Sensei Tips for Layered Process Audits

The following is a Layered Process Audit for the patient appointment process for a physician group practice:

Co-worker Physician Practice Appointment Process	Audit Date:
Observe the process once per day and complete the audit form below. Post results on the dashboard.	

Greeting - Review items below for completeness and accuracy:	**Results**
Is the patient pleasantly welcomed to the practice?	Yes ☐ No ☐
Is the patient proivded the HIPPA consent form?	Yes ☐ No ☐
Notes:	Corrective Action Issued? Yes ☐ No ☐

EMR Update - Verify processes for completeness and accuracy:	
Is the insurance information updated as well as a copy of their Driver's License made?	Yes ☐ No ☐
Are the patient's questions answered and put at ease?	Yes ☐ No ☐
Is the procedure and what is expected meet the patient's expectations?	Yes ☐ No ☐
Notes:	Corrective Action Issued? Yes ☐ No ☐

Collect Payment - Review processes for completeness and accuracy:	
Is the insurance information correct for payment (i.e., co-pays)?	Yes ☐ No ☐
Does the patient check-out in an efficient manner (co-pay, next visit, etc.)?	Yes ☐ No ☐
Does patient require anything at check-out that should have been done during the visit?	Yes ☐ No ☐
Notes:	Corrective Action Issued? Yes ☐ No ☐

Measurables - Review processes for completeness and accuracy:	
Is the patient wait time less than the target of 15 minutes?	Yes ☐ No ☐
Was all the insurance information correct for billing and coding purposes?	Yes ☐ No ☐
Is the patient thanked and pleasantly sent on their way with a "Have a Good Day."	Yes ☐ No ☐
Notes:	Corrective Action Issued? Yes ☐ No ☐

Audit Score = [(11 - (Number of "No" results)) / 11] * 100	**Audit Score:**
(Do not include "No" results for "Corrective Action Issued?" questions.)	_____ %

This part of the Layered Process Audit system was conducted once per shift by a co-worker or peer.

Officer Manager Physician Practice Appointment Process	Audit Date:____
Observe dashboard daily and complete the auidt form below. Post results on the dashboard.	

Co-workder Audit - Review items below for completeness and accuracy:	Results
Is the Co-worker audit being performed once per day?	Yes ☐ No ☐
Are the Co-worker audit results being posted on the dashboard?	Yes ☐ No ☐
Notes:	Corrective Action Issued?
	Yes ☐ No ☐

Corrective Actions - Verify processes for completeness and accuracy:	
Are the Co-worker audits Corrective Actions being identified on the dashboard?	Yes ☐ No ☐
Are the Co-worker audits Corrective Actions being addressed appropriately?	Yes ☐ No ☐
Ave the Co-worker audits Corrective Actions being closed in a timely manner?	Yes ☐ No ☐
Notes:	Corrective Action Issued?
	Yes ☐ No ☐

Audit Score = [(5 - (Number of "No" results)) / 5] * 100	Audit Score:
(Do not include "No" results for "Corrective Action Issued?" questions.)	____%

This part of the Layered Process Audit system was conducted once per day by the Office Manager.

PA (or Doctor) Physician Practice Appointment Process	Audit Date:____
Observe dashboard weekly and complete the auidt form below. Post results on the dashboard.	

PA (or Doctor) - Review items below for completeness and accuracy:	Results
Is the Office Manager audit being performed once per day?	Yes ☐ No ☐
Are the Office Manager audit results being posted on the dashboard?	Yes ☐ No ☐
Notes:	Corrective Action Issued?
	Yes ☐ No ☐

Corrective Actions - Verify processes for completeness and accuracy:	
Are the Office Manager audits Corrective Actions being identified on the dashboard?	Yes ☐ No ☐
Are the Office Manager audits Corrective Actions being addressed appropriately?	Yes ☐ No ☐
Are the Office Manager audits Corrective Actions being closed in a timely manner?	Yes ☐ No ☐
Notes:	Corrective Action Issued?
	Yes ☐ No ☐

Audit Score = [(5 - (Number of "No" results)) / 5] * 100	Audit Score:
(Do not include "No" results for "Corrective Action Issued?" questions.)	____%

This part of the Layered Process Audit system is conducted once per week by the Physician Assistant (PA), Doctor, or head nurse in the practice. Through implementing of this LPA audit system, this physician group practice improved communications and patient/staff satisfaction, as well as reduced wait times by 20% over a 3 month period. LPAs, along with action plans (or PDCAs) for improvements, can help organizations accelerate improvement initiatives and be a positive impact on the bottom-line.

Lean Thinking Statements for the Control Phase

The following Lean Thinking Statement assessment should be done as an individual and, if desired, combined and discussed as a team. If the team leader realizes that many of the items are an issue for certain team members, then maybe a one-on-one with those specific individuals would be appropriate. Or, if a few of the team members have similar concerns over one or two of the statements, then possibly these should be addressed with the team. Continue with open and honest dialogue with the team. As a team member, it is YOUR responsibility to address any of the statements that hinder YOUR individual input to the team's progress. These statements are not to be taken lightly!

Use the 5 Level Likert Scale for the following statements:

> 1 - Strongly Disagree
> 2 - Disagree
> 3 - Neither Agree nor Disagree
> 4 - Agree
> 5 - Strongly Agree

I understand the value of SPC. _____
I participated in creating visual management processes. _____
I believe we should audit our process changes. _____
I believe that Standard Work for Leaders will allow us to better understand expectations from all levels. _____
I believe that if everyone is involved in Layered Process Audits the gains made will be sustained. _____
I can contribute to this team. _____
I am confident in discussing this project with my colleagues. _____
I see the value in this team's approach. _____
I believe I can add value to this team. _____
I believe my ideas will be heard and considered. _____

Total Score: [ ]

If your score is less than 80% (40 points), then more work should be completed before starting another project. Ensure the A3 Project Report Section 8. Follow-Up is completed and shared within the organization prior to starting another project.

Appendix

A3 Project Report Related Questions

> **Project Name:**
> **Process Owner:**
> **Date:**
> **Champion:**
> **Team Leader:**
> **Lean Sensei/Black Belt:**

DEFINE

1. Problem Statement
What data do we have to support the significance of the problem?
What percent of the time are we meeting customer expectations?
What is the impact of the problem on the customers of the process?
What is the "Business Line of Sight" between our strategic goals and dashboards to this particular issue?

2. Current State
What is the value stream or process map, with cycle time and failure data, for this process?
What does the map tell us about the complexity of our process?
What is the feedback from employees/stakeholders on how the process is working for them?
What other data do we need to collect to understand the process?
Can we create a current state with a value stream map (with data)?

MEASURE

3. Improvement Opportunity
How will we know when we have achieved success?
Are there benchmarks or comparative data that we should review?
What should we measure in order to (a) compare "before" and "after" and (b) know how we have made a difference in the process?
Have we identified the wastes?
What does the Voice of the Customer tell us about how we are providing value or meeting expectations?
Can we show our goals using a Balanced Scorecard for the project? (E.g., flow, customer satisfaction, employee engagement, financial impact, etc.)
What does the future state look like?

ANALYZE

4. Problem Analysis

Who will be impacted by changes in this process?

What is the demand for the process – how many requests/patients by hour of the day and/or day of the week?

What is the detailed process flow?

Can we use a Fishbone Diagram to find and show any likely problem areas and their related root causes?

How much waste is there in the process?

Have we asked the "5 Whys" for each step?

Can we show that we have identified the major problems using a Pareto Chart?

Have we used an Impact Map or other tool to prioritize the wastes/problems we will address in this project?

Do we understand the root causes of the problem?

IMPROVE

5. Future State

What gaps exist between current and future states and what changes in the process (PDCAs) should be taken to address these?

What stakeholders will be involved in the action plan?

What is the communication plan?

Can we show a high-level summary of process steps that need to be changed?

6. Implementation Plan

What improvement tools and resources will we need to make the recommended improvements?

What steps need to be taken to accomplish the improvement plan?

Who will take the lead for each step?

What time frame is required? When will the new process be implemented?

What is the training/education plan?

What data will continue to be collected, and how often will it be collected and reported?

How will feedback be obtained from customers and stakeholders?

Can we show a high-level 4 W's of Who (does) What (by) When, and Why for this project?

7. Verify Results
Can we show a chart or graph to display the process "before and after" to answer the question: Is there a difference?
What are the comparative metrics?
Is the new process meeting the target?
Do we have a WWWW to represent any additional work that is needed?
Can we summarize what we have learned from this improvement project?

CONTROL

8. Follow-Up
Has SPC or a Visual Management system been considered to ensure for monitoring improvements?
What have we learned from this project?
How will the results continue to be shared with stakeholders and customers?
How will we share the learnings with others across the system?
What other projects, topics, or issues have we discovered, that should be addressed by follow-up improvement projects?

Lean and EMR

As more healthcare organizations implement an Electronic Medical Record (EMR) system there is a need to design efficient processes that interact with these systems. Lean, and Six Sigma, is a perfect partner to this type of process change. As the saying goes, "we do not want to automate a bad process." Implementing an EMR system, which is the natural progression of IT in healthcare, will not automatically improve the Balanced Scorecard measurements as discussed earlier. However, when processes are analyzed, reviewed, and improved upon utilizing the tools and concepts of Lean and Six Sigma, then and only then will the full benefit of an EMR system be realized and those Balanced Scorecard measurements will improve.

For example, there are many problems inherent with orders in a paper-based process (i.e., illegible writing, misinterpretation of writing, incomplete information, lack of signature, lack of date and time, etc.) that can be considered as "defects" (i.e., wastes) that create rework on the part of clerks, nurses, and other stakeholders. When the order is transcribed into an electronic record, the ordering clinician is responsible for selecting the correct order, modality, dosage, etc. assisted by algorithms built into the program to ensure (for example) that incompatible medications are not selected, or duplicate tests are not ordered. The availability of "Computerized Physician Order Entry" or CPOE, with its clinical decision-making support in the form of built-in pathways or guidelines, is seen as a crucial step towards reducing errors in the ordering process and improving patient safety as the result of clear, correct, and complete orders being delivered.

Likewise, the availability of patient tracking within the Electronic Medical Record (EMR) system, serves as a visual reference. For example, a large monitor can be placed in a central location in ED so that everyone (staff that is) can see what patients are present, how long they have been in the ED, and their status (suitably coded, of course, for HIPAA-required confidentiality). The ability to receive results (i.e., labs, tests, etc.) immediately via the computer system is a superior process to the paper-based flow. In the electronic world, as soon as the department enters and verifies the result, it is available via the computer and an alert is posted to the appropriate caregivers that the results are available for review.

Therefore, the application of Lean and Six Sigma tools should be an important component in the design and implementation of an EMR system.

Lean Facility Design Case Study

Note the before Lean solutions and after Lean solutions in this example. Results were significant in this physical layout change.

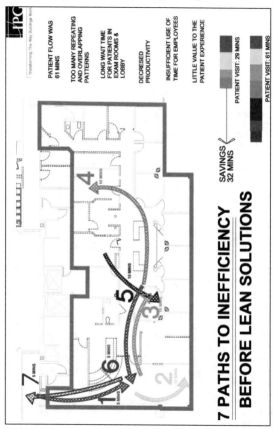

PATIENT FLOW WAS 61 MINS

TOO MANY REPEATING AND OVERLAPPING PATTERNS

LONG WAIT TIME FOR PATIENTS IN EXAM ROOMS & LOBBY

DECREASED PRODUCTIVITY

INSUFFICIENT USE OF TIME FOR EMPLOYEES

LITTLE VALUE TO THE PATIENT EXPERIENCE

PATIENT VISIT: 29 MINS

PATIENT VISIT: 61 MINS

SAVINGS 32 MINS

7 PATHS TO INEFFICIENCY

BEFORE LEAN SOLUTIONS

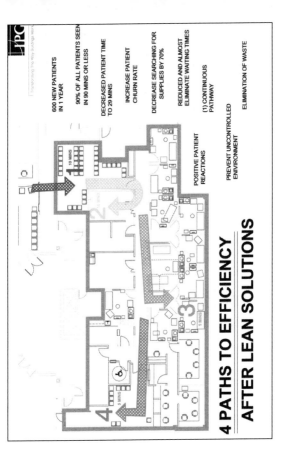

600 NEW PATIENTS
IN 1 YEAR

90% OF ALL PATIENTS SEEN
IN 90 MINS OR LESS

DECREASED PATIENT TIME
TO 29 MINS

INCREASE PATIENT
CHURN RATE

DECREASE SEARCHING FOR
SUPPLIES BY 70%

REDUCED AND ALMOST
ELIMINATE WAITING TIMES

(1) CONTINUOUS
PATHWAY

POSITIVE PATIENT
REACTIONS

PREVENT UNCONTROLLED
ENVIRONMENT

ELIMINATION OF WASTE

4 PATHS TO EFFICIENCY
AFTER LEAN SOLUTIONS

Billing and Coding SWOT Analysis Case Study

SWOT (Strengths, Weaknesses, Opportunities, and Threats) is a business planning method used to evaluate Strengths, Weaknesses/ Limitations, Opportunities, and Threats. The SWOT analysis, if required, typically is completed during the Prepare or Assess Phase (i.e., Define Phase for D-M-A-I-C). It can also be done at any time during the project when this type of information is required.

The Billing Department of a high volume physician practice was having some difficulties meeting deadlines and reducing their Accounts Receivable (A/R) days. The team decided to do a SWOT analysis to ensure the main issues of the department be addressed in the upcoming departmental improvement initiative. Previous attempts to improve efficiencies were met with various levels of success. Basically, within 1 month of the previous improvements, the A/R days were back to where they were before. There was a lack of apathy and buy-in at that time.

The manager of the department wanted more staff buy-in this time around. To get everyone involved and demonstrate a united front moving forward, the manager asked everyone to complete a SWOT analysis on their department. The manager created the following simple matrix to ensure everyone contributed:

Billing and Coding SWOT Analysis Contributors (includes everyone in the department)		
Those who have contributed to SWOT analysis	Position/Role	Completed SWOT
Mary Benjamin	Insurance Verification	Yes
Lisa Hardy	Coder	Yes
Heide Brown	Biller	Yes
Alyssa Rapp	Billing Clerk	On Vacation til 6/22
Suzy Harmon	Biller	Yes
Melissa Marino	Billing Clerk	Yes
Barb Kapler	Insurance Verification	Yes
Dave Roe	Worker Comp	Yes
April Light	Physical Therapy Billing	Yes
Doug Harper	Billing Clerk	Yes
Lisa Rodriguez	Biller	On Maternity Leave
Deanna Troy	Auto Ins Verification	Yes

The manager consolidated the SWOT analysis information received from the staff. The following provides a brief summary of the results:

Criteria Examples:	Strengths	Weaknesses	Criteria Examples:
Capabilities? Unique Selling Points? Resources, Assests, People? Innovative aspects? Price, Value, Quality? Accreditations, Qualifications, Certifications? Processes, Systems, IT? Cultural, Behavioral? Management? Philosophy and Values?	Hard working staff Knowledgeable staff that will work together	Processes and duties change without communication to all staff Lack of training	Gaps in capabilities? Lack of competitive strength? Reputation, presence, and reach? Timescales and deadlines? Reliability of data? Morale, commitment? Leadership? Accreditations? Processes and Systems? Management?

Criteria Examples:	Opportunities	Threats	Criteria Examples:
Market developments? Competitor's vulnerabilities? Industry trends? Technology developments? New markets? Niche markets? New Unique Selling Points? Partnerships? Volumes?	Phones, someone to handle patient concerns on a daily basis. Allow present staff to accomplish their duties and improve patient satisfaction with the same staff.	Ability to balance work loads New reimbursements	Political effects? Legislative effects? Environmental effects? IT developments? Market demand? New technologies? Loss of key staff? Sustainable financial backing? Economy?

The results of this SWOT analysis provided the manager and staff with the beginning of a transformation road map. The team acknowledged their Strengths, then focused on their Weaknesses and Opportunities. A brief meeting with the staff allowed them to sort their Weaknesses using the Impact Map process (pages 133 - 135). This resulted in a focused project list for the staff to work on as they began the A/R improvement project.

Glossary

5S - is a process to ensure physical areas and paper-based or electronic documents are systematically kept clean and organized, assuring employee safety in meeting customer expectations while providing the foundation on which to build a Lean Sigma organization.

A3 Report - is designed to help you "tell the story" in a logical and visual way with reference to a particular subject matter.

Act - the standardization of the improvements after the Check step of the PDCA improvement cycle.

Action Item (AI) Log - used by the team to assign and follow-up on specific actions items agreed to during the project.

Attribute data - a numerical quality that assumes only two values: good or bad, pass or fail, etc. and is measured by counting the frequency of items matching the condition.

Basic process maps (macro level) - identifies all the major steps in a process - usually no more than six steps. They are mostly used for the 30,000 foot view for management review.

Basic process maps (micro level) - examines the process in detail and indicates all the steps or activities that would include the decision points, waiting periods, tasks that frequently must be redone (rework), and any feedback loops.

Brainstorming - a technique used to generate a high volume of ideas with team members' full participation that is free of criticism and judgment within a 5 - 15 minute time period.

Cause and Effect (or Fishbone) Diagram - a graphical display of all the possible causes of the problem. Also known as a Fishbone Diagram.

Check - the verification of the Do implementation step of the PDCA improvement cycle.

Constraint or Bottleneck analysis - the identification of the slowest process step in the product or service being provided.

Continuous flow - the movement of work or a service between processes with minimal or no queue time.

Control Chart - a tool used to determine whether a process is in a state of statistical control or not. Also referred to as a Statistical Process Control Chart, Shewhart Chart, or Process-Behavior Chart.

Defect waste - refers to all processing required in creating a defect and the additional work required to correct a defect.

Define Phase - the initial determination of purpose of the improvement, resources required, and a plan.

Demand Analysis Plots - methods used to understand the pace of customer demand.

Deployment process maps - the visual representation of a process in terms of who is doing the steps. It is conveyed in the form of a matrix, showing the various participants and the flow of steps among these participants.

DMAIC (Define - Measure - Analyze - Improve – Control) - a five step statistical-based problem solving methodology commonly referred to as the D-M-A-I-C process.

Do - the implementation step of the PDCA improvement cycle.

Effective meetings - the efficient and timely organizational communication for a group of people for issues to be discussed, priorities to be set, and decisions to be made.

Environmental waste - any output of a process that negatively impacts the environment.

Facilitator - a person that ensures that everyone attending the meeting stays on task and participates.

Failure Prevention Analysis - a technique that allows the team to anticipate potential problems in the solution before implementing it permitting the team to be proactive to prevent the solution(s) from going wrong.

FIFO - is a work-controlled method to ensure the oldest work (i.e., patient, labs, electronic document, supply items, etc.) upstream (first-in) is the first to be processed downstream (first-out).

Frequency Charts - a method by which to collect, organize, prioritize, and analyze data.

Gantt Chart - a graphical representation of project tasks, sequence, relationships, and time required.

Generation Xers - the people born between 1965 and 1980.

Generation Y (Millenials) - the youngest working generation in the workforce; people born between 1981 and 1999.

Histograms - a method by which to display the spread and shape of the distribution of data.

Impact Map - allows teams to identify solutions most likely to have the greatest impact on the problem with the least effort.

Interrelationship Diagram - an analysis tool that allows a team to understand and identify the cause-and-effect relationships among critical issues.

Inventory waste - excessive piles of paperwork, computer files, supplies and time spent searching for a document.

Kaizen Events - sometimes called "Rapid Improvement Events" or "Kaizen Blitzes" are targeted events conducted by improvement teams to implement improvements quickly in a specific area.

Kanban - a card or visual indicator that serves as a means of communicating to an upstream process precisely what is required at the specified time.

Lean - the tools and concepts derived from the Toyota Production System that minimizes and eliminates waste using Total Employee Involvement (TEI) and a common-sense approach.

Lean Sigma - the combination of the customer-focused efforts of Lean and waste elimination with the quantitative methodology of Six Sigma.

Mass customization - a concept that combines the low costs of mass production processes with the variable output required to meet individual client needs.

Matures (Traditionalist, Veterans, and Silent) Generation - the oldest generation in the workforce and these people were born between 1925 and 1945.

Measure Phase - a full and thorough documentation of the customer needs or market demand for the process being improved as a continuation of the Define Phase.

Mistake proofing - a concept, device, and/or system designed to ensure that it is impossible to make a mistake or produce a defect.

Motion waste - any movement of people, paper, and/or electronic exchanges that does not add value.

Opportunity process maps - the visual representation of the activities that comprise the process and lists differences between value-added and non value-added activities.

Overburdening (or overloading) waste - the unknown capacity or non-productive scheduling of a process.

Overprocessing waste - putting more effort into the work that what is required by internal or external customers.

Overproduction waste - producing some type of work prior to it being required.

Paced Flow - used where customer demand requests are done on a regular or timed schedule.

Pareto Chart - a bar chart format that represents the Pareto principle.

Pareto principle - refers to 20% of the sources causing 80% of the problems.

Performance Dashboard (or Balanced Scorecard) - a visual aid that translates the organization's strategy into objectives, metrics, initiatives, and tasks customized to each group and individual in an organization.

Performance Management - the process of establishing desired performance outcomes or goals, monitoring progress to goals through measurements, and then taking action to ensure success.

Pitch - the adjusted takt time that establishes an optimal and smooth workflow throughout the value stream.

Plan - the define step of the PDCA improvement cycle that determines what will be done, who will do it, and how it will be measured.

Plan-Do-Check-Act (PDCA) - an iterative four-step problem solving process typically used in business process improvement.

Policy Deployment - a methodology to consistently establish, align, communicate, and measure the progress of an organization in achieving their strategic objectives and mission.

Process map (or flowchart) - a visual representation of a series of operations (tasks, activities) consisting of people, work duties, and transactions that occur in the delivery of a product or service.

Project Charter - a document that defines the high level objectives and expectations for an improvement project team.

Project management - the process of establishing, prioritizing, and carrying out tasks to complete specific objectives.

Quality Function Deployment (QFD) - a tool that takes the Voice of the Customer information and turns it into specific and measurable quality requirements that can be used to design improved processes.

Radar Chart - a graphical representation of the values for each listed category along a separate axis that starts in the center of the chart and ends on the outer ring.

Rapid Improvement Events (RIEs) - See Kaizen Events.

Run Chart - a graphical representation of serial data points over time.

Runner - someone that is dedicated to ensure takt time or pitch is maintained and makes "rounds" at specified intervals to pick-up and deliver items.

Scatter (and Concentration) Plots - a graphical representation to study the possible relationship between one variable and another.

Scheduled flow - the method by which orders or demand is identified, and then scheduled for fulfillment at a specific time.

Scribe - the person who records the notes of the meeting; and/or the person who captures the group's thoughts on flip charts, white boards, or the laptop that is being projected on the wall or screen, etc.

Set-In-Order - the part of the 5S step that involves arranging necessary items for easy and efficient access and keeping them that way.

Shine (or Scrub) - the part of the 5S step that involves cleaning everything, keeping everything clean, and using cleaning as a way to ensure all physical areas and electronic files and folders are maintained as they should be.

Sigma (σ) - the representation and mathematical symbol that defines the variation or "spread" of a process.

SIPOC diagram - a tool used by a team to identify all relevant elements of a process improvement project or identified value stream to help ensure all aspects of the process are taken into consideration and that no key components are missing.

Six Sigma (as a business tool) - a structured, quantitative, five-phase approach to continuous improvement and problem solving.

Social waste - the excess time, energy, and resources used that contributes to poverty, injury, malnutrition, etc. as well as the non value-added time spent on account of social media networking.

Sort - the part of the 5S step that involves sorting through the contents of workplace physical and electronic database areas and removing unnecessary items (papers, old manuals, outdated files - both paper and electronic, etc.).

Spaghetti diagram process maps - a continuous line to trace the path of a part, document, person, or service that is being provided through all its phases.

Standard work - a method that establishes and controls the best way to complete a task without variation from the original intent.

Standard Work for Leaders - the guide that prescribes specifics tasks, actions, and time frames for completion of work for a manager or supervisor.

Standardize - the part of the 5S step that involves creating guidelines for keeping the area and electronic files and folders organized, orderly, and clean, and making the standards visual and obvious.

Statistical Process Control - a group of tools used to control and monitor process outputs.

Storyboard - a poster-size framework for displaying all the key information from the Lean Sigma project.

Structured Brainstorming - a defined method in which each team member contributes his/her ideas in order until all ideas are exhausted.
Sustain - the part of the 5S step that involves education and communication to ensure that everyone uses the applicable standards.
Sustainability Metrics - measurements that help organizations identify,

Takt time - defines the pace of repetitive customer demand.
Team champion - the person who has the authority to commit the necessary resources for the team.
Team Charter - the documents the team structure, membership, overall objectives, measures, and resources required to be successful.
Team leader - the person responsible for the day-to-day or week-to-week running of the team.
Team member - the person who is responsible for keeping an open mind, being receptive to change, and contributing their ideas in a respectful manner.
Teaming - a group of individuals working together for a common cause or objective.
Technical representative (tech rep) - the person from IT (or someone with advanced computer application skills) who provides insights into technology tools available and/or makes the team aware of upcoming technology that may impact the team's mission.
Timekeeper - the person responsible for ensuring the scheduled times (start, stop, topics, etc.) are followed.
Total Productive Maintenance (TPM) - the tools, methods, and activities used to improve the machine or equipment availability time.
Transport waste - the excess movement of work to the next process.

Underutilization of people waste - the result of not placing people where they can (and will) use their knowledge, skills, and abilities to their fullest potential.
Unevenness waste - the lack of a consistent flow of inputs/information/scheduled work from upstream processes.
Unstructured Brainstorming - a method in which team members contribute their ideas as they occur (or come to mind) until all ideas are exhausted.

Value stream map - a visual representation of the material, work, and information flow, as well as the queue times between processes for a specific customer demand.
Variable data - data such as length, time, weight, etc. that is measured along a continuous scale of some type.

Visual control - a technique employed whereby control of an activity or process is made easier or more effective by deliberate use of visual signals (signs, information displays, maps, layouts, instructions, alarms, and poka-yoke or mistake proofing devices).

Visual Management - a use of visual techniques that graphically displays relevant business performance data.

Voice of the Customer (VOC) - is a term and method used in business and Information Technology to describe the in-depth process of capturing a customer's expectations, preferences, and aversions.

Waiting waste - the time delay in expecting or delivering some type of work.

Waste - anything that does not add value.

Waste Walk - an activity when project team members visit a process area that is being considered for improvement, ask questions, and then identify the wastes on the current state value stream or process map.

Index

V

W

Y

Notes

Notes

Notes

Notes

Best Selling Books from The Lean Store

Visit *www.TheLeanStore.com* to see these and other best selling books to assist you in your continuous improvement activities:

Lean Office Demystified II - *Using the Power of the Toyota Production System in Your Administrative, Desktop and Networking Environments*
Lean Six Sigma for Service - Pursuing Perfect Service - *Using a Practical Approach to Lean Six Sigma to Improve the Customer Experience and Reduce Costs in Service Industries!*
The 5S Desktop (PC) Pocket Handbook - *Using the Power of the Toyota Production System (Lean) to Organize and Control Your Electronic Files and Folders*
The A3 Pocket Handbook for Kaizen Events - *Any Industry - Any Time*
The New Lean Healthcare Pocket Guide - *Tools for the Elimination of Waste in Hospitals, Clinics, and Other Healthcare Facilities*
The New Lean Office Pocket Guide - *Tools for the Elimination of Waste in Paper-Based and Electronic Workflow Environments*
The New Lean Pocket Guide - *Tools for the Elimination of Waste*
The Simply Lean Pocket Guide - *Making Great Organizations Better Through PLAN-DO-CHECK-ACT (PDCA) Kaizen Activities*
Today's Lean Leader - *A Practical Guide to Applying Lean Six Sigma and Emerging Technologies to Leadership and Supervision*
Value Stream Management for Lean Healthcare - *Four Steps to Planning, Mapping, Implementing, and Controlling Improvements in All Types of Healthcare Environments*

TODAY'S LEAN! SERIES OF BOOKS

Today's Lean! - Learning About and Identifying Waste
Today's Lean! - Using 5S to Organize and Standardize Areas and Files
Today's Lean! - It's All About Workflow
Today's Lean! - Value Stream Mapping for Healthcare

PRACTICAL LEAN SIX SIGMA FOR HEALTHCARE APPS

Practical Lean Sigma for Healthcare - Overview
Practical Lean Sigma for Healthcare - 5S
Practical Lean Sigma for Healthcare - A3 Report

...plus many types of Lean training sets, games, eforms, and books in Spanish and Chinese!